The Ageing of Connective Tissue

The Ageing of

Connective Tissue

DAVID A. HALL

Department of Medicine
University of Leeds
England

ACADEMIC PRESS · 1976
LONDON · NEW YORK · SAN FRANCISCO
A Subsidiary of Harcourt Brace Jovanovich, Publishers

ACADEMIC PRESS INC. (LONDON) LTD
24/28 Oval Road
London NW1

United States Edition published by
ACADEMIC PRESS INC.
111 Fifth Avenue
New York, New York 10003

Library of Congress Catalog Number: 75-46331
ISBN: 0–12–319150-5

TYPE SET BY GLOUCESTER TYPESETTING CO LTD, GLOUCESTER
PRINTED IN GREAT BRITAIN BY CLARENDON PRINTERS, BEACONSFIELD

Foreword

Research into the ageing process and our knowledge of the structure and function of connective tissue have developed side-by-side over the past quarter of a century. I have had the privilege of being engaged throughout the whole of this period in research in both of these interesting fields.

Although I have tried to be as objective as possible, the very fact that I have been so close to much of the research on which I had to report, has resulted in the book developing into one man's very personal picture of what undoubtedly is a very broad field. Both age research and connective tissue studies have been approached on a multi-disciplinary basis, and I make no apology for the fact that I discuss the age relationship of the chemistry, biochemistry, histology, microstructure, physical function and physiology of a variety of different forms of connective tissue, rather than deal in depth with any one topic. It will be immediately apparent that I am not, nor could be, an expert in all these facets of my subject, but one of my aims in undertaking the task of writing this book has been to demonstrate how much can be gained if connective tissues, and more especially their variations with age, are studied from as large a number of points of view as possible.

Throughout my research I have been inspired by two men above all others and also encouraged by contact with the many other colleagues with whom I have collaborated. This book would never have been written had it not been for Professor Sir Ronald Tunbridge who in 1949 introduced me to both connective tissue and to its age variations and Professor Fritz Verzar with whom over the years I have had the privilege of discussing connective tissue studies and of working for the development of international co-operation in experimental gerontology. Although I benefited so greatly from my association with these two doyens of gerontology, neither they nor my other colleagues can be held responsible for the views expressed in this book. It would, however, be wrong for me to fail to mention the following colleagues with whom I have had the pleasure of working and with whom from time to time I have discussed various aspects of connective tissue gerontology: Drs J. W. Czekalowski, T. Davies, S. El-Ridi, J. E. Gardiner, G. N. Graham, P. F. Lloyd, W. R. Miller, C. Murray-Leslie, F. B. Reed, R. Reed; Miss H. Saxl, Drs R. S. Slater, J. D. Teale, I. S. Tesal, J. E. Wilkinson, Professor V. Wright, and the late Drs M. K. Keech, and W. A. Loeven. My thanks are also due to Mrs A. Starkey, who not only takes her place as one of the many technical staff who have helped with my research, but has also typed the manuscript.

David A. Hall   Leeds, May 1975

Contents

Foreword   v

1 Theories of Ageing   1
Definitions   1
Genetically determined phenomena   4
Random error theory   7
Dependent theories of ageing   9

2 Macrostructural Changes in Connective Tissues with Age   13
General structural characteristics of connective tissues   13
Extracellular tissues   21

3 Microstructural Changes in Connective Tissues with Age   67
The X-ray diffraction pattern   67
Electron microscopic evidence for age changes   69

4 Chemical and Biochemical Changes in Ageing Connective Tissues   79
Collagen   79
Elastin   95
Glycoproteins and proteoglycans   136

5 The Metabolism of Connective Tissue   145
Synthesis   145
Degradation   148
Hormonal control of connective tissue metabolism   164

6 Age-Dependent Pathological Conditions in Connective Tissue   173
Vascular diseases   174

References   181

Index   201

1

Theories of Ageing

Definitions

As a preliminary to a study of the ageing of connective tissue it is necessary to define the process of ageing and to settle the meanings of the various terms which will be used to describe the phenomenon.

Age is the state of being elderly, or may also refer to a quantitative measurement of the process of growing old. In the loose terminology of the layman, a person's age refers to the number of days, months and years which have passed since birth. This should correctly be termed *chronological age*. It is a well-known observation that pairs of human subjects of the same chronological age may differ in their appearance and capabilities. In fact, the apparent "age" of their individual organs may vary considerably although they might both have been born on the same day. They may, therefore, be said to differ in their *biological age*, and the notional value to be ascribed to this virtually unmeasurable parameter, may differ from organ to organ and tissue to tissue. A man with a chronological age of 65 may have the carriage and gait of a 40-year old, but have the facial appearance, due to excessive wrinkling and sagging, of an 80-year old.

Although it would be desirable for age to be expressed on all occasions in terms of the biological status of at least one major organ, this is as yet impossible and chronological age is almost universally employed. This results, however, in a considerable scatter in the values which may be obtained for any measurable parameter at any one chronological age, since what is in fact being measured is a series of values for individuals of differing biological age.

In addition to the date of birth (or conception) there is one other point in the male life span, and two in the female, which are fixed for each particular individual. These are the date of attainment of puberty and in the case of the female, the date of the menopause. Comfort (1956) quoted observations by Tanner (1955) in which individual and mean growth velocities over the age range 6 to 18 years were plotted for a group of five boys. When the plots were recorded against chronological age the points of individual peak growth rate were offset over a range of four years (from 10 to 14 years) and a curve drawn through the mean values at each point of chronological age had a particularly broad peak. However, if the curves were plotted against the numbers of years before and after the point of maximum growth velocity (the

1

actual age at which this occurs varying with the age at which puberty is attained), the curves all present a similar profile, and not only does the mean curve have a sharper peak, but the standard deviation of the individual curves around this mean curve is low. Similarly, Hall (1976a) has shown that certain changes which can be observed in the collagen content of the skin of female subjects over the years 45 to 65, can be shown to correlate more closely with the number of years past the menopause than with the chronological age of the individual subjects.

Lifespan, longevity and life expectancy

In many experimental studies on animal populations, assessment of longevity is often employed as a measurement of factors which can affect the ageing process. The number of years which an individual is capable of surviving is related to those changes which occur during life, but only in a secondary sense. Especially in human studies where longevity may not be under the control of a single genetic factor in a complex ageing process, the exact number of years that the individual lives may not bear any direct relationship to the degree of senescence (see below) which is exhibited during the latter years of life.

Life expectancy, although again partially dependent on the response of different organs to the ageing process, is essentially a statistically derived function, which is in no way related to changes in the structure or function of the organs and tissues of the individual.

Senescence

This is defined as a deterioration in function and structure. When it can be subjected to measurement, the values obtained are an assessment of decreased viability and increased vulnerability to external and internal insults. The study of senescence entails the examination of a group of physiological processes, all working towards the deterioration of a state of adult vigour which may represent the peak of achievement.

Criteria of ageing

Strehler (1962) suggested that any physiological phenomenon must meet four criteria before it can be unequivocally considered to be a component of the overall ageing process. These four criteria are those of:
1. Universality
2. Intrinsicality
3. Progressiveness
4. Deleteriousness
Every ageing phenomena must be identifiable in all members of one species, although the degree to which they effect the functioning of the organism may

well vary from individual to individual. Thus for baldness to be classified as a true age phenomenon, it must be demonstrated that during life at least all male subjects lose some portion of the number of viable hair follicles with which they are endowed at maturity. This is in fact probably true of females as well, although, at its greatest extent female baldness is far less apparent. This is only one of the variety of phenomena which although age related, are sex-linked, but this apparent sexual specificity should not necessarily mean that they are excluded from the lists of factors concerned in the overall ageing process. The concept of *intrinsicality*, introduced by Strehler as a criterion of the ageing process, implies a restriction of acceptable ageing factors to those changes which are of endogenous origin. Although it is patently obvious that subjects of different age react differently to external stimuli, it is the response rather than the stimulus which is the age related factor. Thus the differential effect of ultra-violet radiation on the physical and chemical properties of the proteins of the skin of young and elderly subjects (p. 115) is dependent on the changing susceptibility of the skin collagen to irradiation rather than to any effect which is directly attributable to the ulta-violet light itself.

All true ageing phenomena develop *progressively*, and for this reason it is necessary to distinguish between those effects which have a higher incidence above a certain age, but which develop rapidly and those which develop progressively with increasing age. Although the underlying susceptibility of the tissue or organ concerned may alter with age, the acute episode which finally brings a catastrophic change to the notice of the patient or to his physician, is not a typical ageing phenomenon. Thus underlying changes which develop with age within the coronary vessels may precipitate a myocardial infarction, but the terminal occlusion itself which finally cuts off the blood supply to the particular segment of heart muscle, although more prevalent in late middle and old age, cannot be regarded as an age determined incident. On the other hand the development of atheroma and the repair processes which result in the production of fibrous plaques on the intimal surfaces of the major vessels (p. 178) although not strictly universal in occurrence, may be regarded as marginally age dependent.

The fourth of Strehler's criteria – *deleteriousness* – is a concept the acceptance of which by workers in the ageing field has caused considerable controversy. Thus it has long been appreciated that the collagen of the new-born animal is rich in monomeric protein chains, but that as the animal ages these monomers become linked with one another by the formation of cross-linkages (p. 90). Verzar (1963) and Bjorksten (1958), on the basis of observations on the strength and stability of collagen from animals of varying age, have propounded theories of ageing which ascribe many of the physical characteristics of old age to the increased rigidity of collagen molecules which contain an increasing number of cross-links. More recent studies have demonstrated that in the main the numbers of cross-linkages only increase during the period of maturation (Bailey, 1969) and over the past few years a number of suggestions have been made (Jackson, 1973a; Hall, 1968a) which indicate that the effect of cross-links is merely to ensure that the collagen is increasingly fitted for the role it has to play in the tissues of which it forms a part. Therefore, if the concept of *deleteriousness* is accepted for all aspects of the ageing process, the existence of cross-linkages alone cannot be regarded as the sole cause of true age effects. Degradative changes must ensue when senescence sets in, and although the degree to which this occurs may be dependent on the degree of cross-linking (p. 114), the cross-links themselves merely have a secondary role to play in ageing.

Genetically determined age phenomena

In 1962 and 1972 the journal *Chemical and Engineering News*, which might be expected from the nature of its readership to have little vested interest in the promulgation of one particular theory of ageing at the expense of another, published two special reports on the human ageing process. At the beginning of the second one (Sanders, 1972) it is stated that "The causes of human ageing are almost as much of a mystery today as they were 10 years ago". Although this is a true assessment of the situation, the last decade has seen the polarisation of the mystery in one or two directions. Firstly, attempts by workers to implicate a single lesion in the whole complex of metabolic processes, as being the prime factor in initiating observable age changes, have given way to a realisation that ageing may in fact be induced by a number of different mechanisms operating simultaneously. Different organs and tissues of the body may age in completely different ways, and it would be wrong to assume that the approach of any one group of research workers is more likely to provide an answer which will be universally applicable in the search for a unique factor, than is the approach of any other group. If this book had been written ten or fifteen years ago, the writer would have had to attempt to show how one or more of a number of apparently unconnected theories could explain the ageing of connective tissue. At the present time it is possible to group together the many theories which were current fifteen years ago, into two major divisions which are essentially covered by the concepts of:

1. Programmed ageing theory
2. Error theory

It is generally accepted that ageing is governed to a major extent by genetic factors. For instance Pearl and Pearl (1934) were able to show that human longevity can be predicted with a fair degree of accuracy from the sum of the ages at death of the two parents and four grandparents of the subject under consideration. Similarly an examination of genetic factors must help to explain why elephants live for 60–70 years, rats for up to 4 years, tortoises

150 years, fruit flies 40 days and butterflies only 24 hours (Comfort, 1956). The maintenance of a mean life span for any one species must be determined by a group of genetic factors which are transmitted from parent to offspring. It is possible that the genetic make up of each organism may contain certain genes which control the "genetic clock" determining the speed at which the metabolic processes are performed, and the length of time which elapses before death occurs. Hayflick (1965) demonstrated that fibroblasts from foetal connective tissue would multiply satisfactorily *in vitro*, until 50 divisions had occurred. Although it had long been assumed that cell lines were immortal when cultured outside the body, these cells died after 50 mitotic divisions. In contrast, cells from similar tissue of a 20-year old man were only capable of 20 divisions before death occurred. Hayflick suggested that the cells stopped subdividing and died not because of any external factor, but on account of an intrinsic factor within the cells themselves. This factor might consist of a lethal gene especially programmed for release after a given number of cell divisions or it might be that the lethal nature of the gene only becomes apparent at second hand. If the degree of deterioration of DNA or RNA which occurs throughout the life span of the cell strain can normally be repaired by enzyme systems produced by the cells under the control of a group of genes, then the failure of such a repair process after a given number of cell sub-divisions, due to the repression of these genes, would have a similar effect in the long run as that of a direct-acting lethal gene.

In the living organism, the growth of cells comes under the control of tissue hormones, which either repress mitosis or by their absence permit cell division to proceed. In this way tissues may survive in the body for far longer than they would *in vitro*. Krohn (1962) has demonstrated by serial transplantation of skin tissue from mouse to mouse, that a single piece of skin can survive for a period which is many times longer than the life span of the animal from which the tissue was originally removed. Studies of the changes which take place in cell lines, either *in vitro* or *in vivo*, permit information to be obtained concerning the deterioration in organ function which occurs in the period preceding death. It is of greater importance, especially in so far as human subjects are concerned, to be able to ascertain which factors control the deterioration of bodily function during the latter half of life than to be able to determine the nature of factors which control life span. It can be assumed that certain lethal genes, or genes which control nucleic acid repair, are specific for those tissues which although important are not directly responsible for the maintenance of life. During the development and differentiation of such a tissue different gene loci along the length of the whole nucleic acid molecule in the chromatin strand, are rendered capable of transcription by the removal of an appropriate repressor substance. The control of the production of these repressor substances is mediated by regulator genes, and it is at this level that the overall control of cellular function may be located.

The programmed alteration of function of any single tissue or organ depends on the controlled transcription of individual gene loci, during the period when any one parent cell produces its offspring. During differentiation the changes are such as to produce cell clones which are capable of developing a tissue which is increasingly more suited to the task it has to perform. If programmed degeneration is to account for deleterious changes in organ function with increasing age, the individual cells of the ageing tissue, as they sub-divide, must produce daughter cells which are less capable of providing the enzyme systems required for dealing with the cell's surroundings, or daughter cells which are so markedly different from their parents as to be recognised as alien by the defence mechanisms of the body.

The production of daughter cells which, although capable of survival, have a different enzyme make up from their parents will result in an alteration in the function of the organ of which they form a part. This may take the form of de-differentiation, if the cells revert to a primitive state, or degeneration if the differentiation is no longer positive with respect to increasing tissue function. On the other hand if patently alien cells result from an unnatural sub-division, the new cells will react with humoral or cellular anti-bodies, and will be eliminated from the organism. This will bring about a reduction in the total number of cells of a given cell line with a concomitant loss of activity of the organ concerned. Either result would be deleterious to the functioning of the organ and could engender those types of degenerate changes which are apparent in old age.

Evidence for programmed changes such as these are scanty, although the late Dr Howard Curtis reported (Curtis et al., 1966) the incidence of an increasing number of abnormal chromosomes in mice and dogs as they aged. More direct evidence which could explain the apparent failure on the part of cells to continue to differentiate and adapt themselves to the changing condition associated with middle and advanced age, stem from the experiments of von Hahn (1964), who studied the binding of histones to DNA in the livers and thymuses of young and old rats and cattle. He observed that histones show an increased and firmer binding to DNA as the animals age. These histones may represent the repressor substances which control the release of specific gene loci for transcription, and an excessive degree of permanency in their attachment to the nucleic acid will prevent the cells undergoing further differentiation, and the presence of greater amounts of bound protein may result in the DNA of the daughter cell being incapable of taking part in even that degree of transcription of which the DNA of the parent cell was capable.

Although it is patently obvious that some, at least, of the ageing phenomena are programmed, and hence genetically determined, alterations in the

DNA, its breakdown, repair or degree of attachment to the accompanying histones cannot explain all the observed senescent changes. One of the major points which confirms this is the failure of agents such as ionising radiation or radiomimetic drugs, which damage DNA, to alter the life span of intact organisms to a comparable degree. For this reason much of the current research on the primary ageing lesion has transferred from the nuclear nucleic acid, DNA, to the cytoplasmic one, RNA.

Random error theory

The genetic information which is handed on from parent cell to daughter cell is neatly programmed in the nuclear DNA and altered appropriately by the repression of some gene loci and the de-repression of others, to enable cell differentiation to proceed. The daughter cell makes use of this information by translating it into the appropriate RNA code, which, in the form of *messenger* RNA, in association with particulate bodies, the ribosomes, acts as a template on which proteins can be synthesised. Individual amino acids, phosphorylated and in the form of a complex with their specific activating enzyme are picked up by a molecule of *transport* RNA, which is itself individually programmed for that particular amino acid and carried to the ribosome when their particular neucleotide codes in the m-RNA molecule are in association with either a single ribosome or a ribosome cluster. Peptide linkages are then formed between each newly arrived amino acid and the previously synthesised portion of the protein chain, and this process continues with the addition of amino acids, in the number and order prescribed in the m-RNA code, until the whole protein has been built, and a code neucleotide which instructs the completion of the polypeptide chain is reached. The production of each individual protein requires the involvement of enzyme systems at many stages. Synthetases control the translation of the DNA code to the appropriate RNA template, and activating enzymes prepare the individual amino acids for peptide formation. All these various enzymes, being protein in nature are synthesised in the same way. Orgel (1963) pointed out that an error introduced into the synthetic pathway of any one of the enzyme proteins, would affect subsequent cycles of protein production, and could result in an accumulation of errors which might impair cellular function and might ultimately be lethal.

This concept of the retention and amplification of error syntheses which, having once been introduced into the protein synthetic pathway has received a considerable amount of support, although experimental verification is as yet confined to a limited number of laboratories. Holliday (1972) has shown that the production of a single error in a unicellular organism, or in mammalian cells, by the provision of a slightly abberrant intermediate fluorouracil results in the production of an increasing proportion of the inactive form of certain enzymes. This phenomenon of increasing denaturation in enzyme systems is a well-known concomitant of ageing (Holliday and Tarrant, 1972).

Three difficult questions remain to be answered, however, before the error theory can be fully accepted. Firstly it is necessary to define the primary causative agent which introduces the first error; secondly, one has to answer the question; if the reproduction and amplification of an error is so widespread, how do organisms resist an overall disruption of their metabolic processes relatively early in life? Thirdly, if the errors are random errors, how can such a theory meet the first of Strehler's criteria (p. 2) since it might be assumed that each individual would age in a different fashion?

One possible answer to the first question involves the introduction of the hypothetical concept of naturally occurring mutations, or spontaneous error induction. If one considers the possibility of a mutation inducing the first error, one is in effect returning to the suggestion that nuclear DNA is involved, since a mutation is defined as a faulty transcription of DNA during mitosis. Danielli (1956) suggested that ageing and death might be due to the accumulation throughout life of non-lethal somatic mutations. However, such changes would of necessity be restricted to actively dividing cells, and it is apparent that much of the ageing process takes place in tissues, the metabolism of which is controlled by cells in their post-mitotic phase. Orgel's suggestion moved the site of the initial error one stage nearer to the final product of cellular metabolic activity, by assuming that it was just as possible and even more probable, that an error would occur in the translation and synthetic pathways as at the transcription level. No biological system can be expected to carry out its functions correctly for ever, and the feed-back amplification effect which would result from production of only a single error during the synthesis of one of the enzymes involved in such a process ensures that the number of errors required may well be quite small.

On purely mathematical grounds the insertion of an error in the synthetic pathway could result, in a relatively short time, in the production of second, third and fourth generation error proteins. Is there then an answer to the second question posed above? Any explanation of this apparent paradox must involve the immunological defence mechanisms of the body. Just as was suggested in the section above, in which programmed age phenomena were considered, the majority of the aberrant proteins which will be produced as the result of a single error, are adequately controlled by cellular and humoral immunological processes. Only a limited number will escape this net, either because their degree of deviation from normality is not sufficient to warrant antibody formation, or because by pure chance the presence of an error protein is associated with an error in the synthesis of the specific humoral or cell surface antibody.

It is much harder to find an acceptable answer to the third question. The relatively similar fashion in which all members of one species undergo ageing would at first sight, appear to discount the possibility that ageing is in fact due to the accumulation of random errors. It would appear most likely that the ageing process is a biphasic phenomenon, and that any factor which depends on the introduction of self-perpetuating faulty syntheses may merely act within a framework defined by a programmed ageing process. Hence, the general age changes which can be observed in a species such as; progressive loss of muscular activity, changes in organ function, cerebral atrophy and other universally apparent phenomena leading inexorably towards death at a certain age, cannot be avoided by any normal member of the species. Superimposed on these are the individual changes which slightly alter the age incidence of the various ageing effects, and make possible the existence of individuals who have aged more rapidly or who show marked differences in the rates at which their various organ senesce.

Dependent theories of ageing

The theories of ageing discussed in the previous section, by their very nature can only be applied at a molecular level. They are therefore only applicable to ageing as it is observed at the tissue, organ or whole organism levels, in so far as they may explain the reason for the occurrence of these phenomena. Various of the earlier theories which were introduced to explain in a more pragmatic fashion some of those aspects of senescence which are apparent at higher levels of organisation may be reintroduced here therefore, since they represent obvious developments of the programmed and random error theories of ageing.

Cellular fall out

This phenomenon has long been suggested as a causative factor in ageing. Actual counts of the number of cells in representative samples of brain tissue led Andrew (1938) to suggest that the number of brain cells lost per day might assume quite astronomical levels. This work has been expanded to include other tissues, and although some of the methods of sampling may leave much to be desired, evidence has accumulated over the past ten years on the basis of which the concept of increased cell death with ageing, has been justified. Franks et al. (1974), however, have measured the DNA, and protein contents and the total number of nuclei in the whole brains of members of a colony of ageing mice (Strain C57BL). No significant differences were found in a series of animals ranging in age from 5 to 158 weeks old. By using entire brains, all sampling error is removed, and this may, therefore, indicate that some of the suggestions based on the microscopic examination of serial sections of relatively restricted regions of the brain may be heavily biased.

As far as connective tissue is concerned the cellular concentration, even in relatively young adult animals is quite low. It might appear therefore, that changes in such a small number of cells would be immediately observable. No one has reported a reduction in fibroblast count, during the ageing of an adult animal however, although Hilz et al. (1963) have demonstrated a 50% decrease in the cellular population of rat aorta confined to the first two months of life. It would appear that one must look elsewhere for the reduction in cellular activity which accompanies ageing.

Changes in enzyme levels

The enzymes synthesised by a given line of cells depend on the status and function of the tissue of which the cells form a part. Mitotically active cells are rich in DNA and RNA synthetases. Cells which provide energy for tissue or organ function are rich in enzymes of the glycolytic pathways, and those which are engaged in protein synthesis, in many instances contain an array of enzymes of the transaminase group which are essential for the synthesis of the amino acids required for protein production. At the other extreme, those cells which have catabolic function produce high concentrations of either generalised or specific proteolytic enzymes.

Estimations of enzyme levels in various tissues, throughout life have shown that although some remain roughly constant, others may either rise or fall. (Meyer et al., 1940; Bourne, 1957; Kirk, 1959; Mandel, 1961; Bertolini, 1962; Ghiringhelli et. al., 1963; Zorzoli, 1969 and Wilson, 1973). Those enzymes which suffer a reduction in activity with age may well do so as the result of errors occurring in the synthetic processes by which they are produced on the cytoplasmic ribosomes, but rising levels of activity would at first sight appear more difficult to explain on this basis. It is, however, possible to account, not only for rising levels of enzymic activity, but also for those situations which exist in the case of certain enzyme systems, whereby the activity appears to pass either through a peak or a trough during middle age (Silberberg and Lesker, 1973; Wilson, 1973).

Many enzymes exist in tissues and organs in close association with inhibitors which control their activity. These inhibitors are in most cases also protein in nature, and their synthesis is therefore controlled on the ribosomes in a similar fashion to that which determines the production of the enzyme for which they are specific. Assuming that inhibitor activities modify the absolute effect of the enzyme by subtracting an appropriate proportion from the uninhibited enzymic activity thus providing a value which may be referred to as the effective or apparent enzyme activity, all the various curves which describe the changes in effective enzyme activity with age can be broken down into two curves. These represent age changes in enzyme levels and inhibitor levels respectively, and as can be seen from Fig. 1 all can be represented by the difference between two falling curves. These two curves, can both be ascribed to the accumulation of errors in the synthesis of the enzyme and the inhibitor proteins, although the composite curve may rise or reach a peak value in middle age. The curves in Fig. 1 are all hypothetical, but to take a particular case as an example, Silberberg and Lesker (1973) have reported that the level of β-glucuronidase activity in the articular cartilage of the male guinea pig rises during the first $2\frac{1}{2}$ years of life, and falls thereafter. This shape can arise if a curve recording an inverse power relationship between inhibitor and age is subtracted from one which describes a linear relationship between enzyme and age.

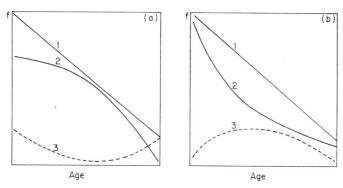

FIG. 1. Theoretical curves demonstrating how maxima and minima can be produced in curves relating effective enzyme activity to ageing. (a) Linear fall in absolute enzyme content of a tissue coupled with an increasing rate of loss of inhibitor results in minimal effective activity at intermediate ages. (b) Linear enzyme loss coupled with a decreasing rate of inhibitor loss results in an intermediate maximum value.

Hormonal control of the ageing process

It has long been believed (Brown-Séquard, 1889) that age changes in tissue, and the dysfunction of certain organs, can be reversed or prevented by the administration of extracts or suspensions of cells from organs which synthesise hormones. Brown-Séquard's observations have been supported by Steinach (1920); Voronoff (1920, 1929) and Niehans (1954), all of whom have employed tissue extracts in controversial "rejuvenation" procedures. Although these workers in general employed glandular cell preparations, they suggested that it is the cells rather than the hormones which they contain, which are responsible for the tissue changes which they claim to observe. There is, however, a considerable body of evidence (cf. Asboe-Hansen, 1966) which indicates that the hormones themselves may have a direct action on tissue proteins especially those which are constituents of the connective tissues.

Since it is well appreciated that the hormonal balance of the mammalian body suffers a number of variations with age, it is to be expected that some at least of the observed degenerative processes may be associated with these hormonal changes. Good (1958) claimed that the phenomenon of ageing was due to a slowly developing hypo-function of the thyroid, and such age-regression in the activity of this gland has subsequently been demonstrated (Pittman, 1962). However, even ageing thyroids react to the normal extent when stimulated with thyroid stimulating hormone, and hence it might be assumed that the control of the ageing process may lie in the pituitary rather than the thyroid. The effect of hypophysectomy on connective tissue meta-bolism is discussed in detail below (p. 168). Variations in corticosteroids have also been observed with increasing age, and this may be either the cause or the result of involuntary processes associated with senescence.

2

Macrostructural Changes in Connective Tissues with Age

General structural characteristics of connective tissues

The various forms of connective tissue are all characterised by a massive development of intercellular substance. The cells which exist are separated from one another and scattered throughout the fibrous matrix, and the relative proportions of cells and matrix vary with the function of the individual tissue. In some types of tissue, especially the loose connective tissue which is the most generalised form of this constituent of the body, the cells are quite numerous, in others such as tendon they are few in number and even when the nuclei are stained, appear insignificant in relation to the closely packed fibres which make up the majority of the intercellular matrix.

All species of connective tissue arise from differentiation of the mesoderm, and in particular from the mesenchyme of the middle germ layer. The mesenchyme develops in the early stages of embryonic life by the migration of cells from the sclerotome or ventral portion of the primitive mesodermal segments. At this stage the whole mass consists of an array of cells, processes from adjacent surfaces of which form a network which entrains a homogenous fluid substance rich in protein. Later this fluid becomes more viscous with the appearance of mucoid material and in this ground substance appear the fibres which ultimately constitute a large proportion of the intercellular substance.

Initially they lie in close proximity to the cellular processes, but as the tissues develop they become separated from the cells, and either align themselves in bundles (the collagen fibres) or with the later appearance of the elastic fibres form a network throughout the intercellular space. This embryonic tissue then differentiates further into one or other of the adult forms of connective tissue with the development of larger amounts of fibrous protein and more numerous types of cell. Some of the tissues such as tendon, vascular wall, skin and ligament develop in such a way as to become essentially a solid fibrous mass; the fibres being separated by relatively small quantities of mucoid-rich ground substance, and the cells amounting to only a very small proportion of the whole. In the loose connective tissues which lie subcutaneously and attach the skin to the underlying tissues, or form the stroma of the organs and the adventitial borders of the large blood vessels, the essential

13

identity of embryonal connective tissue is maintained. There is a predominance of interstitial substance, but the fibres are not bound together in bundles. The major portion of the intercellular space is amorphous ground substance, and the tissue as a whole is easily distorted and displaced. Other tissues such as cartilage consist of similar proportions of fibrous protein and polysaccharide, but the nature of the latter component is such that the tissue assumes a rigid although pliable conformation. Specialised tissues such as Wharton's Jelly in the umbilical cord are essentially devoid of fibrous masses, and the polysaccharide provides a homogenous jelly-like consistency. In bone the proteinaceous matrix becomes mineralised to provide the rigid structures required for skeletal stability. All these variations in constitution are dependent to a marked extent on the function of the tissue concerned, and since connective tissues provide the connecting, supporting and protecting structures of

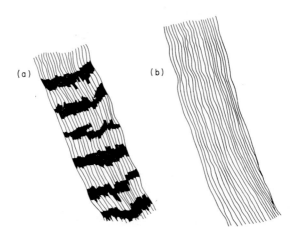

FIG. 2. Diagrammatic representation of tendon fibres illuminated with polarised light. (a) Unstretched, showing alternate regions of anistropy and quenching. (b) Stretched, slightly, showing complete orientation and loss of quenching effect.

the body, the number and organisation of the fibrous elements in the intercellular matrix determines the suitability of each tissue for its specialised function. Thus in tendon which has to resist longitudinal forces, collagen fibres, which are essentially inextensible, are arrayed parallel to one another along the axis of the tissue (Fig. 2). In the aortic wall, where the major forces are those of distension, and in the skin where two-dimensional extension occurs over joints, the same relatively inextensible collagen fibres are converted into an extensible structure by being aligned in layers or bundles at an angle to one another (Fig. 3). Forces which distend such networks in the

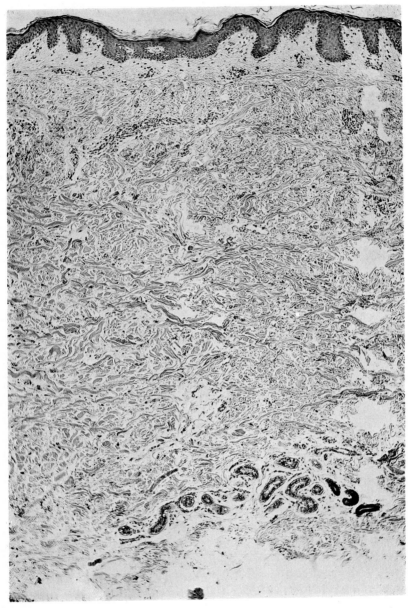

FIG. 3. Section of human skin stained with Weigert's elastica stain. (×60)

aorta or act in the plane of the crossed bundles in the skin, tend to rotate the fibres and as the inextensible elements turn relative to one another so as to lie in parallel arrays, appreciable extension of the tissue as a whole can occur. The simultaneous presence of elastic fibres in these latter types of tissue assists in the return of the network of collagen fibres in its unstretched conformation. Ligaments, on the other hand, which have to withstand a greater degree of extension, are rich in elastin fibres, the relatively small amounts of collagen merely acting as a strengthening element to prevent over-extension.

Connective tissue cells

There are a variety of cellular bodies which can be identified in connective tissue, although only a limited number of all the cells which can be identified in such tissues are an essential part of the structure.

Fibroblasts. The most important and numerous cells in all forms of connective tissue are the fibroblasts. These are large flat branching cells with extensive processes protruding from adjacent cells. They often appear in close proximity to fibre bundles and at least one of their major functions is the synthesis of the proteins from which these fibres are formed. Fibroblasts are found in all forms of connective tissue, and they are virtually the only cellular type present in closely packed tissues such as tendon.

It was originally believed that collagen and elastin fibres arose spontaneously in the intercellular matrix completely without cellular intervention (Virchow, 1871; Maximow and Bloom, 1953). This was, however, disproved in the early years of the present century, and the fibroblast was later shown unequivocally to be the cell type responsible for collagen fibre formation (Jackson, 1968). Similar doubts were expressed concerning the synthesis of elastic fibres (Doljanski and Romlet, 1933) and it has only recently been shown that fibroblasts are also involved in synthesis of this form of fibre as well (Bourne, 1951). During the development of the human embryo, or during tissue regeneration following trauma, the synthesis of collagen fibres precedes that of elastic fibres by an appreciable period (Okajima, 1957) and it has still not been ascertained which particular factors determine the nature of the protein to be synthesised at each sequential stage in the synthesis of these tissue components. At each phase in the development of the tissue, the cellular type associated with the newly synthesised protein, be it collagenous or elastic, is the fibroblast. It may be that two forms of fibroblast which are indistinguishable from one another by normal histochemical procedures, may exist side by side in those tissues which will ultimately contain both collagen and elastin. One of these cell types may be predominant during the early stages of tissue development, resulting in the exclusive production of collagen, whereas at a later stage some as yet unknown humoral or physical stimulus may induce the second line of cells to commence protein synthesis resulting in the development of elastic fibres. Conversely the stimulus may act within a single cell line inducing an alteration in the nature of the protein which these cells synthesise, by repressing the gene locus responsible for collagen synthesis, and de-repressing that which controls elastin synthesis. Similarly the production of glycosaminoglycans or lipids which occur in specialised tissues such as cartilage and vascular wall may be brought about by the activation of specialised cell lines which have hitherto remained dormant, or by the differentiation of part of the fibroblast population.

Histiocytes or macrophages are found in all loose connective tissues. They are irregularly shaped with processes which are usually shorter and blunter than those of the fibroblasts, and the nucleus is usually smaller. As their name implies they are actively phagocytic, ingesting any dye or pigment injected into the living organism, and can thus be identified in connective tissues by *intra vital* staining (Evans and Scott, 1921). Their function would appear to consist in the removal of tissue debris following trauma or when tissue remodelling necessitates the degradation of already existing tissue proteins, and hence they may be very active in aged or diseased tissues.

Mast cells. These are probably the next most important group of cells in connective tissues, being responsible among other things for the production of the sulphated polysaccharide heparin, which is released into the tissue fluid following the rupture or extrusion of metachromatic granules present in their cytoplasm. Since collagen fibres are capable of initiating thrombus formation by interaction with platelets in the plasma, the simultaneous presence of heparin-producing cells may represent a homeostatic factor in connective tissue, since heparin inhibits a later stage in the clotting reaction.

Pigmented cells. Specialised connective tissues, such as the choroid and the iris of the eye, and the corium of dark-skinned races, contain cells which are pigmented. The cytoplasm of these cells contains varying amounts of the brown or black pigment melanin. These pigment granules are synthesised by the cells themselves from tyrosine, and are not phagocytosed after synthesis in other sites in the body.

Intrusive cells. In addition to these various cell lines, which are native to the connective tissues, many wandering cells from the blood and lymph streams are often present. They may include lymphocytes and eosinophilic and neutrophilic leucocytes which are attracted to the connective tissue by stimuli originating either within or without the organ concerned.

Changes in cell population and functions with age. The number of cells present in all but a few very specialised connective tissues is very small, and hence it might be expected that assessment of changing cell populations could easily be made by visual or automated scanning of stained tissue sections. In fact the very paucity of the cell populations militates against this, especially since cells are not evenly distributed throughout the tissue. Hence, sections may be cut for histological examination which appear to have a concentration of cells greatly in excess of the true population, whereas others may appear to be abnormally devoid of cells. This is a phenomenon which is true of all tissue components which are present in small concentration and are irregularly dispersed (cf. distribution of elastic fibres in skin p. 41). It has therefore, proved necessary to devise methods for the estimation of cellular populations which rely on the biochemical assessment of a relatively constant cellular component such as DNA. The accuracy of this measurement however, is dependent on a number of factors, not all of which are conducive to accurate assessment of cell numbers. Thus tissues containing fewer cells with larger nuclei may appear to have as high a DNA content as tissues with a larger number of micro-nucleate cells. Measurements of alterations in cell population can only be justified therefore, if it is assumed that the type of cell remains constant throughout, and must be confined to single tissues which have become fully differentiated. Secondly, measurement of a given DNA content does not indicate that all the nuclei containing this nucleic acid are present in living cells. Although dead cells will be removed by their phagocytic neighbours, an appreciable but variable number at any one count may have died so recently as not to have been engulfed and digested. Similarly erroneous estimations of native cellular concentrations in tissues, can result from determinations of DNA made on tissues which are suffering massive degradation or are involved in some inflammatory process. During the destruction of tissue or following the degradation of plasma proteins which are present in the tissue, polypeptide chemotactic agents are released, which attract polymorphonuclear leucocytes and macrophages into the tissue. The function of these cells is the removal of tissue debris and the ultimate return of the tissue to a healthy state, but their presence can outweigh the native cell population, and can result in grossly inflated DNA levels. Ross and Benditt (1964) have demonstrated the presence and function of intrusive monocytes in wound repair. As these cells ingest tissue debris, they develop into mature macrophages, and if the lesion becomes chronic, as may often occur in elderly subjects, will remain in these sites (Carr, 1973) thus affecting the native cell counts for long periods after the apparent healing of the wound.

Allowing for these restrictions to its use the measurement of DNA can demonstrate marked changes in cellular populations with increasing age. For instance Hilz et al. (1963) (Fig. 4) have reported marked changes in the DNA content of the ageing rat-aorta during the first 12 months of life, followed by a very slow fall over the succeeding 2 years. Silberberg and Lesker (1973) have reported changes in cell content in guinea pig articular cartilage from 2 weeks to $5\frac{3}{4}$ years. In this case the dramatic fall observed in rat aortic tissue by Hilz *et al.* is not apparent during the first 12 weeks. In fact there is a 45% rise in DNA content over this early period of growth followed by an 88% fall during the rest of the first year of life. Thereafter the DNA level remains constant.

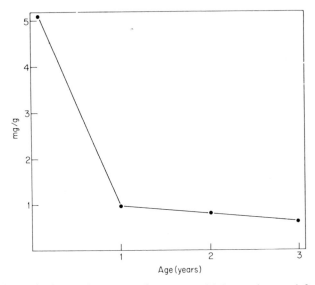

FIG. 4. Change in the DNA content of rat aorta with increasing age (after Hilz *et al.*, 1963).

In the human subject, quantitative biochemical DNA analysis has been carried out by Lindner and Johannes (1973) on the aortic wall. Although the graphical representation of their findings appears to be directly comparable with that for rat aorta presented by Hilz *et al.* (1963) they did not in fact obtain values for subjects younger than 10 years of age, hence the shape of the curve may be uncertain for these early years. However, on the basis of all these findings one may assume that with the exception of a short uncertain period in infancy, the cell population as assessed by estimations of DNA content falls for a number of tissues with advancing age. If one wishes to assess the number of *active* cells in a tissue and its change with age, it is necessary to measure a synthetic function of the tissue as a whole. Junge-Hülsing and Wagner (1969) have in this way studied the activity of cells in the rat aorta, heart and skin, in the synthesis of collagen, total cardiac protein, enzymes responsible for certain aspects of ground substance synthesis (sulphate activating enzymes) and the synthesis of these ground substance sulphated mucopolysaccharides themselves. They measured the uptake of radioactivity from administered ^{14}C-proline into the hydroxyproline fraction of rat aortic collagen, of ^{35}S-sulphate into sulphomucopolysaccharides of rat skin and of ^{14}C-leucine into the total protein and sulphate activating enzyme protein of rat heart. They expressed the "age" of their animals in terms of their weights, and demonstrated between 62 and 90% loss in the incorporation of amino acids and sulphate as the rats "aged" from 50 to 250g. The fall in activity of heart cells with a mean value of 70% is appreciably less then the reduction in activity of cells in either of the other two tissues, in both of which the fall with age is of the order of 90%.

Buddecke *et al.* (1973a) have reported similar measurements for the aortic glycosaminoglycans of ox aorta, measuring the uptake of ^{14}C and ^{35}S into the chondroitin sulphate, dermatan sulphate and heparan sulphate components of the tissue from cattle aged from birth to 13 years of age. An exponential fall in the uptake of radioactivity similar to that reported by Junge-Hülsing and Wagner, for rats was observed for all the individual glycosaminoglycans.

If cellular population measurements based on DNA estimations, and cellular activity assessed in terms of incorporation into a tissue component of a radioactive tracer, are combined to provide values for the activity of the individual cells, varied results are obtained, depending on the tissue being examined. Lindner and his colleagues have performed this type of study on the incorporation of ^{35}S-sulphate into the glycosaminoglycans of rat skin and aorta (Lindner and Johannes, 1973) and rat cartilage (Lindner, 1973). Both activity and the cellular population of the aorta fell with age; by about 85% in the first year of life and at a slower rate thereafter. However, since Lindner and Johannes report DNA levels in terms of mg/g of *wet tissue* but the activity in terms of cpm/100 mg *dry weight* the amount of activity per cell falls by about 25% in the first year and at a slightly more rapid rate up to 3 years of age. The ratio of activity to DNA remains essentially constant throughout life in the case of rat skin, and in cartilage, after a 50% fall in the first year, remains constant for a year and then rises sharply (by 33%) in the third year of life (Lindner, 1973). Similar late rises in the cellular activity of guinea pig cartilage have been reported by Silberberg and Lesker (1973) but here the change-over from a falling to a rising curve occurs at 3 months. These workers studied a different group of enzymes which are also involved in glycosaminoglycan metabolism namely α-glycerol-P-dehydrogenase, phosphofructokinase, hexokinase and aldolase. They rose 7, 10, 10 and 12 fold respectively between 3 and 36 months.

On the basis of the error theory of ageing it is not difficult to explain those cases in which there is a fall in cellular activity. Holliday (1972) and Lewis and Tarrant (1972) have shown that the provision of abnormal amino acids to a cellular system which is actively engaged in the synthesis of enzyme protein results in the production of appreciable amounts of inactive enzyme. Any error introduced into the synthetic pathway would have a similar effect; lowering the overall cellular activity of the system.

Extracellular tissues

Tendons

Studies on the ageing of connective tissues can be said to have started with the observations made by Verzar and his colleagues (Verzar, 1963) on the physical properties of rat tail tendon. Among other reasons for his use of this tissue, was the ease with which the individual tendon fibres can be removed from the animal immediately after death, with the minimum degree of dissection. Verzar and Hüber (1958) studied the appearance of the rat tail fibre under oblique illumination, and reported marked alterations during the first month of life. Helical striations could be observed and these became more definite as the animal matured. Reed (1957) also observed a helical configuration in finer collagen fibrils, when these were examined in the electron microscope and the existence of such structures at various levels of tissue organisation may indicate the progressive development with age of a helical configuration extending from the macromolecular level of the tropocollagen molecule through to the intact fibre. At ages above four months, the helical structures observed by Verzar in the rat tail tendon remained unchanged.

Under the action of heat, collagen fibres can contract by as much as 30%. This phenomenon has been known for an appreciable time, and the temperature at which the thermal denaturation occurs – the shrinkage temperature (Ts) – has proved of considerable use in the leather trade in the assessment of the degree of tannage (Gustavson, 1956). The shrinkage of tail tendon can be recorded even more easily than is possible for skin in view of the ease with which separate fibres can be removed from the tissue as a whole and Banga (1966) has demonstrated that a cross helical structure can be observed in chemically or thermally contracted fibres, when they are examined in polarised light. The appearance of these helices is associated with the release into the surrounding medium of a certain proportion of soluble collagen and Hall and Reed (1957) reported slight changes in the range of values for shrinkage temperature between a young age group (7–9 years) and an old group (89 years) and this was confirmed by Brown et al. (1958). Using rat tail tendon, Chvapil and Jensovsky (1963) and Radhakrushnan et al. (1964) also demonstrated a rise with increasing age. Elden (1965, 1966), however, was unable to confirm this, and suggested that since it has been shown that the melting temperature of collagen from a variety of species is proportional to the sum of the proline and hydroxyproline contents of the molecules, it would not be expected that there would be such change in Ts with age in any one species, or even among the vertebrates as a whole, since the amino acid composition of collagen changes only slightly with age within a species or class.

Verzar (1957) demonstrated that the contraction of collagen fibres under the action of heat exerts a force, which is a function of the age of the animal from which the collagen is derived. The simplest method for the obervation of such changes in contractile forces is to measure the contraction of rat tail

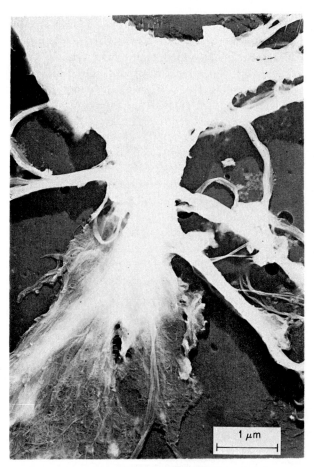

1 μm

FIG. 5. Electron microscope study of metacollagen prepared by the action of Ringer's solution at 60 °C on human skin collagen.

tendons of differing age at elevated temperatures under differing applied loads (Verzar, 1955). The greater the applied load, the less the contraction and the higher the temperature needed to achieve it. The application of a sufficiently heavy load can inhibit the contraction of a young fibre completely, but as soon as the load is removed contraction proceeds to completion (about 70%) if the temperature is above 60 °C. Brocas and Verzar (1961) also studied the isometric forces induced in a fibre held at constant length during the elevation of temperature and showed that, whereas tendon fibres, approximately 0.14 mm in diameter, from 3- to 4-month old rats exert a contractile force of about 1 **g** when heated to 60 °C, similar fibres from 30-month old animals exert at least 10 **g** force.

Banga *et al.* (1956) have shown that a similar age-controlled contraction occurs when fibres are subjected to treatment with 40% potassium iodide solution at room temperature, and Chvapil (1959) has reported a comparable effect with sodium perchlorate. If the fibre is maintained in the same environment, either of temperature or chemical solution, it relaxes and returns slowly to its original length (Chvapil, 1959). When fully contracted, the fibre is elastic, has completely lost its typical microstructure as observed under the electron microscope (Fig. 5), stains with elastica stains, and can be dissolved by elastase but no longer by collagenase. This modified collagen, has been called by a number of different names: metacollagen (Banga *et al.*, 1956), collastromin (Tustanovski *et al.*, 1960), and pseudoelastin (Gillman *et al.*, 1955a, b, Hall, 1968a), although it is possible that these various terms have been ascribed to substances which may differ slightly in their properties.

The effect of age on the tensile properties of tendon

Tendon is a relatively simple tissue, in which the major fibrous protein constituent is collagen, and the collagen fibres lie parallel to one another in an ordered array. Viidik (1966a, 1968) has defined tendon as being essentially an "ideal" material since it approaches the Hookean form of extension, in which there is a constant ratio between stress and strain over appreciable ranges of both extension and load. Stress is defined as the applied force per unit cross-sectional area (W/A) and strain as the degree of deformation per unit original length $(\Delta L/L)$. The ultimate effect of applied stress is the rupture of the fibres composing the tissue, and finally with the total collapse of the tissue sample. Although measurements of the load at break are purely of academic interest, since under normal circumstances the tendon works well within a quarter of this loading (Elliott, 1965; Harkness, 1968), the determination of the ultimate tensile stress has proved of interest to experimentalists, as an extension of studies on other naturally occurring and man-made fibres. Viidik (1966a) and Yamada (1970) have tabulated many of the reported figures and show that they lie between 45 (Stucke, 1950) and 125 newtons/ mm² (Cronkite, 1936) and that there is little change with age (Yamada, 1970).

The mechanical characteristics of a Hookean elastic element can be symbolised by a spring (Element I in Fig. 6) and the slope of the straight line relating stress and strain is the factor E – Young's Modulus. There is no time element in this function. As soon as the load is applied the tissue is stretched, and theoretically the removal of the load results in the complete return of the specimen to its original dimensions.

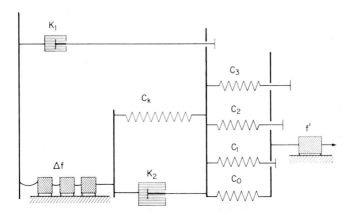

FIG. 6. Schematic representation of the rheological properties of tendon. K_1 and K_2 are elements with the properties of dash pots, C_k, C_3, C_1, C_2 and C_3 springs, the series C_0–C_3 coming into play one after the other, and Af and f′ are dry frictional elements (after Viidik, 1968).

Fung (1967) has pointed out that the determination of a value for Young's Modulus for tendon, as for many other biological entities is possibly pointless, since it increases from zero at negligible load, to relatively high values at high levels of stress. Morgan (1960) and Ridge and Wright (1966a, b) have suggested a power law equation to explain the relationship between stress and strain, and Viidik (1966b) has devised a method for the determination of a so-called "modulus of elastic stiffness" for that portion of the stress/strain curve which is essentially linear. It is, however, the very fact that only a portion of the curve is even quasi-linear, and that the shape of the curve varies with age, that necessitate the evolution of a more complex description of the factors which make up the relationship between stress and strain in the tendon.

There are two ways in which the extension of the naturally occurring fibre can deviate from the Hookean form of extension typical of the simple spring. If a viscous element is introduced as in the compression or extrusion of a Newtonian liquid, the relationship between stress and time will remain constant, i.e. the relationship will be linear as long as the applied stress is retained at a given level. If the applied load is considerable the strain will be minimal during the early stages in its application, and movement of the tissue will only occur as the period of application lengthens. This element is represented in the formalised stress/strain diagram by a dash pot, in which a piston moves in a viscous fluid. Just as the removal of load from a dash pot piston does not result in the immediate return of the piston to its original position, the presence of a viscous element in an extensible material prevents its rapid return to the original dimensions as soon as the stress is withdrawn.

Spring and dash pot may be coupled either in parallel (the so-called Kelvin element) or in series (the Maxwell element). The former permits the ultimate redistribution of a load, initially absorbed by the dash pot, throughout the spring, whereas the spring in the Maxwell element is immediately strained in response to the load, but an additional element of strain builds up in the dash pot with time. When the load is removed, the stress in the Kelvin element decays exponentially to zero, whereas that of the Maxwell element decays instantaneously by the amount appropriate to the strain in the spring, leaving the strain in the dash pot at the level it had reached due to its own slower extension.

Viidik and Mägi (1967) have suggested that a non-linear spring function can best be described by considering a series of springs arranged is parallel so that individuals come into action gradually, spring 2 only being stressed when spring 1 has been strained to a certain extent, and so on.

The final element which can be introduced to explain some of the phenomena observed when stretching non-Hookean materials, is *plasticity*. This is the major factor responsible for hysteresis, i.e. the performance of different stress/strain curves during the loading and unloading portions of an extension cycle.

The stress/strain curves which Viidik attempts to explain by the interaction of these various "ideal" factors were first obtained for tendon by Wertheim (1847) and more recently by a number of groups of workers (Rigby *et al.*, 1959; Morgan, 1960; Wright and Rennels, 1964; Viidik and Mägi, 1967; Elliott, 1967). Viidik employed a method for the explanation of the shape of these curves which demonstrated a close analogy with the array of idealised elements, as developed above. This method had originally been devised for biological materials by Alexander (1962) for the sea anemone body wall) and by Sedlin, 1965 (human bone).

Viidik (1968) observed that successive stress cycles on the same sample became steeper, and moved towards the right, i.e. the tissue became stiffer. On the basis of this he suggested that tendon might consist of the following elements: a Kelvin element in series with an array of springs which come into action serially, and a small dry frictional element to account for the plasticity of the tissue. This described the major curvilinear portion of the relationship (Fig. 7), but the first part of the rising curve after the toe is produced by a dash pot and a further frictional element which consists of individual elements combined in series to produce a build-up of friction with a resulting strain hardening effect.

When in a relaxed state the individual collagen fibres are wavy, and the toe of the stress/strain curve represents the period during which these fibres are straightened out (Rigby *et al.*, 1959; Elliott, 1967; Abrahams, 1967; Viidik and Ekholm, 1968).

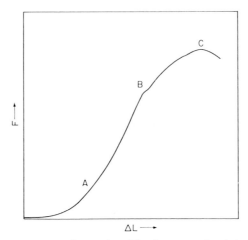

FIG. 7. Load/Extension curve for tendon. The foot, to point A is caused by slippage of fibres over one another. The section A–B represents the actual extension of the tendon. Failure occurs between B and C and the tendon ruptures at C.

The aortic wall

Morphological changes in the vascular system which are strictly attributable to ageing alone, are often difficult to disentangle from other changes which are due to the degenerative processes of arteriosclerosis. Over the past twenty years many attempts have been made to analyse the degenerative changes in vascular tissue, but without any conspicuous success. In fact a number of workers have now accepted that those generalised aspects of arteriosclerosis which comply with Strehler's concept of *progressiveness* (Strehler, 1962), may be regarded as being true ageing phenomena and deserve to be studied as such (Milch, 1965), whereas acute conditions such as those associated with the later stages of coronary insufficiency which precipitate the development of an infarction, cannot. Those degenerative processes in the arterial wall which meet the requirement of being progressive in development, will therefore, be included in this chapter, or in chapter 6, even though they may be regarded by some (Craciun, 1973) as not being representative of a notional *normal physiological ageing process*.

Physical properties. With increasing age the dimensions of the major blood vessels alter. Wellman and Edwards (1950) measured aortas from subjects ranging in age from the first to the tenth decade, and Ehrich *et al.* (1931) made a similar study of the various coronary vessels. The aorta increases in circumference from below 30 mm to above 60 mm over this period, the increase being rapid until growth ceases and then continuing at a relatively steady rate of approximately 0.25 mm/year. The vessel wall increases in thickness from 1.2 mm to 1.65 mm during the first four decades, and then remains roughly constant for the remainder of the adult life of the animal. Since the diameter and the thickness together provide a measure of the cross-sectional area of the tissue, it is not surprising, in view of the observations reported above, that Wellman and Edwards also observed a considerable increase (7 fold) in cross-sectional area with age. Part of this increase will no doubt be due to the laying down of more tissue, but part at least must be due to irreversible distension of the vessel.

During development and subsequent degradation, the physical properties of the aortic wall alter markedly. Burton (1967) quotes a definition of arteriosclerosis which includes the term "loss of elasticity and contractility", and such a description may also be applied to the effects of ageing on the physical properties of the artery wall. The tensile strength of aortic elastic fibres is of the order of 1×10^6 Nm^{-2} (Burton, 1967), whereas that of collagen is 3×10^7 Nm^{-2} (Buck, 1951; Krafka, 1937). The collagen fibres are not all aligned parallel to one another in the wall (see below), and therefore, the collagen fibres are not stretched until an appreciable degree of distension has occurred. The *moduli* of *linear extension* (Young's Moduli) for these two components of the tissue are: elastin – 3×10^5 Nm^{-2}/100% elongation and collagen – 1×10^8 Nm^{-2}/100% elongation (Burton, 1967). This value for collagen has been calculated for this hypothetical degree of extension for comparison with the elastin figure, since the elongation at break of a collagen fibre is far less than this. The extensibility of elastin is therefore at least 300 times (Burton, 1967), and possibly up to 10 000 times (Hall, 1966) greater than that of collagen. The smooth muscle fibres on the other hand are between 30 and 50 times more extensible than elastin, depending on whether their extensibility is measured in the relaxed or the contracted state (Burton, 1967). In normal young aorta, therefore, the major factor which imparts resilience to the tissue is the elastic fibre component, the smooth muscle being far laxer, and the collagen, on account of its topographical distribution, only being brought into play rather in the nature of a check rein, at the extremes of distension. Roach and Burton (1959) have stretched rings of tissue cut from aortas of varying age, have measured the tension induced per unit length and have plotted these values against the percentage increase in the circumference of each ring (Fig. 8). In the case of subjects below the age of 10 years, 100% increase in circumference can be attained by the application of a tension of less than 0.3 N/cm. The necessary tension for the production of even smaller degrees of extension increases with increasing age until in the 80–100 year age group, 40% extension requires 1.5 N/cm. Even at this advanced age, however, the first 20% extension (due to the redistribution of the collagen bundles) can be accomplished by the application of a tension of 0.3 N/cm. To

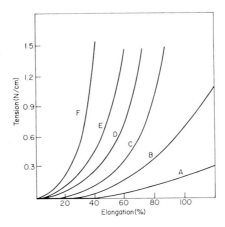

FIG. 8. Curves relating the elongation of rings of human aortic tissue to the tension exerted to extend them; ten year age groups. A, mean age 5 years; B, 15 and 20 year groups with means of C, 30; D, 50; E, 70; F, 90 years.

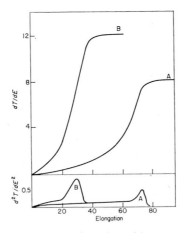

FIG. 9. First and second differentials of tension with respect to elongation calculated from the 30 and 90 year groups (Fig. 8), (after Roach and Burton, 1957). The areas under the d^2T/dE^2 curves are proportional to the numbers of collagen fibres being stretched, indicating that whereas half the fibres are stretched, when the tissue has been extended 60% in the case of the younger group, the same proportion are stretched when 25% extension of the old tissue has been achieved.

account for these age changes Roach and Burton (1957) calculated the rate of change of tension with elongation (the first differential of the curves in Fig. 8), and then the rate of change of this function with elongation (the second differential). They deduced that the area under the peaked curve, which resulted from plotting this second differential against the extension, is indicative of the number of collagen fibres which are under stress, and that the position of the peak is dependent on the proportion of the total number of fibres which are actually undergoing extension. They deduced from their observations that ageing and atherosclerosis are characterised not only by an increase in the collagenous fibre content of the arterial wall, but also by a tightening up and removal of slack in these fibres. Thus at 30 years of age some 50% of the fibres are stretched when the total elongation of the tissue is 60%, whereas at 90 years of age the stretching of 50% of the fibres only results in a 25% extension (Fig. 9).

The intima. The walls of the elastic arteries consist essentially of five separate layers. The immediately periluminar layer is cellular and consists of flattened endothelial cells which are polygonal in shape when viewed from the lumen of the vessel, and lie in close association with one another, being devoid of any demonstrable intercellular cement. In youth, this endothelial layer is relatively homogenous in structure, but numerous cells of varying shape and size appear in elderly aortas (Cotton and Wartman, 1961).

The endothelial layer lies on a basement membrane, which varies in thickness from virtually nil in the case of infants to a thick sub-endothelial layer consisting of a fine network of collagen and elastic fibres, reticulin and smooth muscle, interspersed with histiocytes and fibroblasts all enmeshed in an amorphous mass of ground substance proteoglycans. The development of this layer occurs gradually with age. Moon and Rinehart (1952), who studied the changing rate of synthesis of connective tissue fibres in this region of the aorta with increasing age, by visual assessment of histological preparations of proximal segments of coronary arteries, reported a 13-fold increase in fibrous involvement of this area, between the first and the eighth decade. The ground substance proteoglycans can be stained with Alcian Blue or with metachromatic dyes, and increasing concentrations can be observed in all immediately sub-endothelial layers with increasing age. In general, the changes which occur, and which can be observed in the light microscope have been admirably recorded by Milch (1965) who in turn lists thirty-seven papers in which observations on age related changes in the histological appearance of the inner layers of the aorta are reported.

The internal elastic lamina. Moving outwards from the lumen of the vessel, beneath the endothelium and the sub-endothelial fibrous layer lies the third layer, the internal elastic membrane or lamina. Whether this should be classified

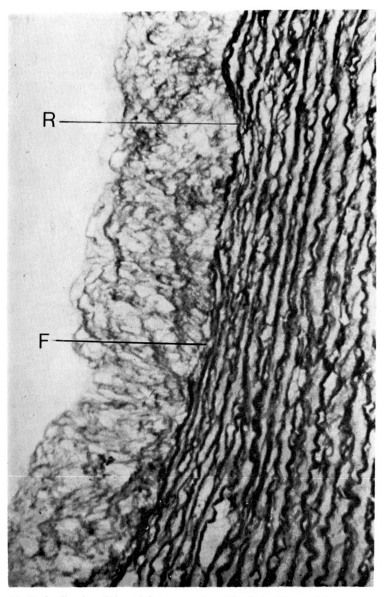

FIG. 10. Reduplication (R) and fragmentation (F) of the internal elastic lamina of the aorta of a rat in which an atheromatous plaque had been induced by the administration of a butter-rich diet. (×300)

as a separate membranous entity lying between the intima (endothelial cells and sub-endothelial layer) and the outer areas of the wall (the media and the adventitia) or conversely should be classed as the outer element of the intima or the inner element of the media is probably only of academic interest. It can be shown, however (p. 100), that the susceptibility of the elastin content of the intima to attack by the enzyme elastase, differs from that of the medial elastic tissue hence, it may be assumed to be either a component of the intima or a specialised layer acting as a medio-intimal junction, in a similar fashion to the elastica staining and elastase susceptible dermo-epidermal junction in the skin.

In early youth the intimal membrane appears as a single convoluted layer of elastica-staining material, but with increasing age the single lamina becomes fragmented and reduplicated until it assumes a much broader cross section with anastomoses between adjacent layers (Fig. 10). Moon and Rinehart (1952) report that the degeneration of the internal elastic lamina runs completely parallel to the fibrosis of the intima.

The media. Outside the internal elastic membrane lies the media, which consists of concentric lamellae of elastica-staining material from the inner and outer surfaces of which fine elastic fibres protrude to anastomose with those from adjacent lamellae (Ayer, 1964). In between pairs of elastic lamellae lie smooth muscle cells, but as the distance from the lumen increases, these are increasingly interspersed with collagen fibres which lie at an angle to the axis of the vessel in helical configuration; fibres in pairs of adjacent inter-lamellar spaces being offset on opposite sides of the axis. It is this three-dimensional weave that permits the distension of a structure containing essentially inextensible collagen fibres (p. 27). Each elastic lamella is virtually structureless when stained with one of the specific elastica stains and viewed in the light microscope. If sections are cut tangentially to the cylindrical tubes of tissue so that semi-circumferential sections of a number of lamallae are included in each field (Fig. 11) it can be seen that the lamellae are not continuous sheets, but are perforated, numerous fenestrations being apparent in each layer. The function of these orifices will be considered later. The medial lamellae of new-born and infant animals (Fig. 12) are highly contorted when viewed in cross section. In life the vessel wall is slightly distended even at rest, due to the mean intravascular blood pressure, but on death the stagnant volume of the blood is less than the volume associated with the mean flow rate during life, and hence the vessel wall contracts, producing the contracted effect observed in the young human aorta in Fig. 12, and also reported for the rat up to 18 days of age by Berry *et al.* (1972). In older tissues, even the relaxation resulting from removal from the body does not return the lamellae to a convoluted state (Fig. 12). They are retained in a tighter

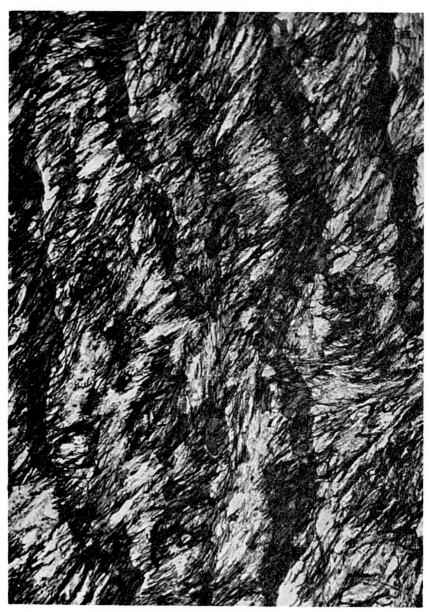

FIG. 11. Section through human aortic wall cut at a tangent to the circumference. Each elastic lamella is sectioned at an angle. Fenestrations and inter lamellar fibrils can be seen clearly. (×500)

orientation, as can be deduced from the studies on the tensile properties of the tissue performed by Burton. Wood (1954) has suggested a reason for a similar change in the spatial distribution of elastic fibres which can be observed in the ageing ligamentum nuchae, and his theoretical explanation may also account for the variation in appearance observed in Fig. 13. In point of fact, the effect

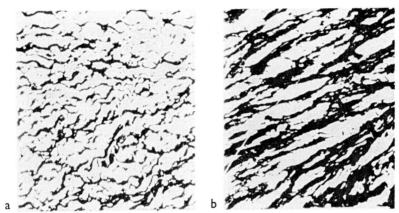

FIG. 12. Comparison of young (a) and old (b) human aortas, showing highly convoluted fine medial lamellae in youth, and broader straighter lamellae in older tissue. (×400)

observed in the ligament is the exact opposite of that which is observed in the aorta, the collagen fibres showing a more convoluted alignment in older ligamentous tissue, whereas in older aortas it is the elastic lamellae which are straightened out. Wood suggested that the inextensible collagen fibres which lie in between the elastic fibres tend to slip past one another during repeated extension cycles, and that when the tissue of an elderly subject is allowed to relax the elastic fibres, as they return to their original length, cause the collagen fibres to assume a twisted appearance since they are unable to slide back over one another. In the aorta, similar relative movement of the collagen fibres during repeated distension cycles may result in their maintaining the elastic lamellae in a partially extended state, even when the internal pressure on the vessel is removed after death. This is in complete agreement with the explanation of the changes which are observed in the diameter of the vessels with increasing age and the shape of the tension/extension curves in Fig. 8.

The thickness of each elastic lamella also increases with age. Berry et al. (1972) have observed an increase in lamellae thickness of from 1 μm to 10 μm between birth and 22 weeks in the rat. Wolinsky and Glagov (1967) have pointed out that the number of lamellae in the aortic media varies with the aortic diameter, so that the tension per lamellar unit, remains constant. This tension is in fact a constant value of 20 ± 4 Nm^{-1}, irrespective of species. The increasing number of lamellae, which Berry *et al.* (1972) have reported as rising from a mean value of $5\frac{1}{2}$ per individual media in the thoracic aorta of a one week old rat, to 7 at 20 weeks, and from 3 to 5 over the same period in the abdominal aorta, must be assumed to be due to the increasing diameter of the aorta in this first 5 months of life.

The adventitia. This outer layer of the aorta contains the *vasa vasorum*, the minor vessels which supply that portion of the vessel wall which is too far removed from the intima to be supplied directly by diffusion from the lumen. Wolinsky and Glagov (1969) have suggested that the improved blood supply to the vascular tissue which is provided through these minor vessels permits structural modifications to occur resulting in the addition of an increasing number of elastic lamellae. The rat is without *vasa vasorum* but Berry *et al.* (1972) believe that a certain degree of remodelling is possible, and that although the total number of lamellae may not increase after the first rapid growth phase, the total number of fine fibrils which protrude from the surface of the lamellae and which anastomise with those from adjacent lamellae to form a three-dimensional network, and which surround and penetrate the bundles of collagen fibres lying in the interlamellar spaces, increases not only during the first 20 weeks of life during which the full complement of lamellae are produced, but also throughout the later months of adult life. The function of these fibrils has not been fully elucidated, but their presence in increasing numbers undoubtedly adds to the resilience of the three-dimensional network, if they do in fact have the full elastic properties of normal elastin.

Smooth muscle. The inner interlamellar spaces contain a larger cell population than most connective tissues. The majority of these cells are representative of the cell species to which the name smooth muscle cell is given. The smooth muscle adds an active contractional force to the passive contraction of the elastic tissue. In young aortas the muscle cells which are spindle shaped are closely packed in between the collagen fibres and lie with their axes roughly parallel to the elastic lamellae between which they lie. With increasing age the muscle cells rotate until their axes lie more closely parallel to the radius of the vessel, and cytoplasmic processes may occasionally be seen to penetrate through the holes or fenestrations in the elastic lamellae (Fig. 13). There is considerable evidence that during the formation of atherosclerotic plaques, smooth muscles cells may migrate in relatively large numbers into the sub-endothelial layer, where they undergo metamorphosis into the lipophages which are recognised, following the removal of lipid during normal fixation processes, as the foam cells of the atherosclerotic plaques (Leary, 1941). Murray *et al.* (1966) have also observed differentiation of smooth muscle cells following arterial damage. As the healing of a surgical incision progresses, smooth muscle cells from the uninjured tissue on either side of the wound assume some of the structural characteristics of fibroblasts and appear to migrate into the wound area, where they give rise to collagen fibres which assist in the closure of the wound space. Similar differentiation of foam cells which have themselves probably derived from smooth muscle cells originally present in the media has been reported during repair processes in atherosclerosis (Branwell, 1963). Organ cultures of lipid-rich tissue excised from the region of an atheromatous plaque in the aortic wall remain viable, but lipid filled, if grown on normal or lipaemic plasma. If, however, plasma containing heparin is administered to the culture, clearing factor is released, the cells are purged of lipid, and differentiate into fibroblasts which produce collagen fibres. This may account for the late appearance of fibrous plaques in sites where repair processes have been initiated to deal with pre-existing lipid deposits.

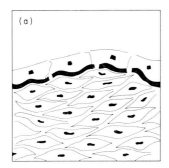 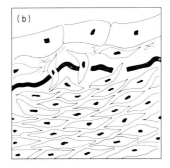

FIG. 13. Diagrammatic representation of (a) young and (b) old aortic wall. Fenestrations in the internal elastic lamina are penetrated by smooth muscle cells with advancing age (b). Fine elastic-staining fibrils can be seen near the terminal processes of these cells which have penetrated into the sub-endothelial region.

Elastic degeneration. In many ageing aortas, and especially in the regions beneath arteriosclerotic plaques, the intima and one or more elastic lamellae may disappear (Fig. 14). The outlines of the elastica staining elements first become blurred, and then the whole lamella dissolves. These changes are directly comparable with those which can be observed when elastic tissue is treated with the pancreatic enzyme elastase (Fig. 15) and it may therefore be assumed that the disappearance of elastica staining material from the aorta with advancing age, may be attributed to the increasing effectiveness of elastase in this tissue. The changing mode of action of elastase on elastic tissues of different age is dealt with in detail elsewhere (p. 100) suffice it to say at this point that the original observations of Balo and Banga (1949) regarding the relationship between elastase action and at least the later stages of

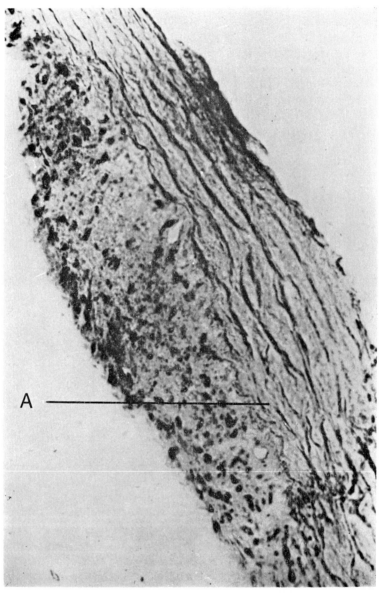

FIG. 14. The digestion (A) of medial lamellae occurring spontaneously beneath an artificially induced plaque. (×300)

arteriosclerosis appears to be fully acceptable, notwithstanding the polemical arguments which have surrounded these topics since their original paper was published.

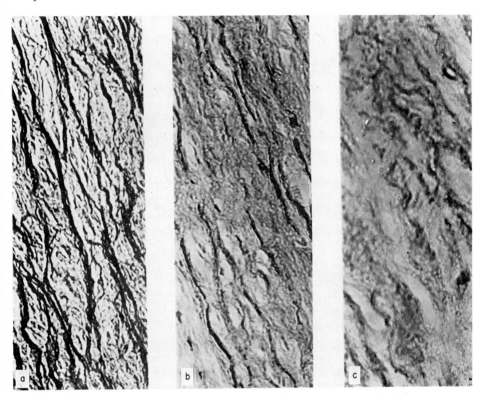

FIG. 15. The effect of elastase *in vitro* on sections of human aorta, stained after treatment with Weigert's elastica stain. (a) Untreated tissue; (b) 2 h incubation; (c) 12 h incubation. ($\times$400)

Calcification. At a relatively late stage in the ageing process, the connective tissue elements of the vascular wall may become highly calcified. Numerous workers have studied the phenomenon of aortic calcification (Gazert, 1898; Baldauf, 1906; Haythorne *et al.*, 1936a, b; Lansing *et al.*, 1948; Blumenthal *et al.*, 1950; Buck, 1951; Kanabrocki *et al.*, 1960; Bolick and Blankenhorn, 1961; Yu and Blumenthal, 1963). Yu (1967), has summarised these studies and added his own observations. The calcium content of human aorta, after a slight fall during the first 10 years of life, rises 40-fold over the next 8 decades. Wells (1933) had observed that the elastic fibres showed a predilection for the uptake of calcium. Histochemical techniques, especially that of microincineration, when compared in serial sections with staining techniques which are specific for elastin, enable the location of the calcium phosphate to be unequivocally identified as being co-terminous with the elastic lamellae (Fig. 16). If the elastic elements are isolated from the aorta, the calcium content of the elastin may be shown to increase even 60-fold between 10 and 90 years of age. The presence of such large masses of calcium phosphate in a crystalline form (Yu, 1967) in the wall of the artery results in a marked alteration in the physical properties of the tissue. In many elderly subjects this results in the formation of the so-called pipe-stem vessel. Not only does the presence of calcium phosphate suppress the resilience of the elastic elements, but the cellular activity of the medial tissue is also reduced so that *de novo* synthesis of collagen and elastin is almost completely inhibited. Yu and Blumenthal (1963) have studied the ultra-microscopic appearance of collagen and elastin isolates obtained from aortas of varying age and have demonstrated that calcification occurs within an amorphous layer which overlays both collagen and elastin, and which increases in amount with increasing age. This material which is less electron dense than the elastic fibres themselves appears to be identical with the pseudoelastin which has been reported by Hall and his colleagues (Hall *et al.*, 1955; Keech, 1955) as being present in increasing amounts with increasing age (cf. p. 10). Whether this material is degenerate collagen, as has been suggested by Hall (1968a) or degenerate elastin as inferred by Yu (1967) is not as yet resolved, it has some of the properties of elastin. Yu suggests that during its degeneration, elastin may unfold, this exposing a "large number of polar centres", which may act as nucleation centres for the deposition of apatite. Since "young" elastin does not contain more than 5% of polar amino acids, the 2-fold increase which Lansing *et al.* (1951) reported in "old" elastin (p. 108) cannot be accounted for by unfolding alone, and even if large portions of the non-polar regions of the elastin molecule are lost during degeneration, the ratio of degenerate to normal elastin would have to be quite high to provide the 10% polar amino acids present in "old" elastin. Hall (1967) has in fact suggested that the pseudoelastin which he believes to be derived from collagen has 31% polar content which represents some 90% of the polar content of collagen.

This increase in the polar amino acid content in the region of the elastic lamellae, will provide centres to which calcium can become attached. The first calcium atom may be bound to the protein by the formation of a co-ordinate shell around its nucleus, with electrons which are partly donated by ionised carboxyl groups, and partly shared with hydroxyl or amino groups. This firmly bound calcium atom may then form one corner of the calcium phosphate crystalline lattice, which results in the precipitation of apatite crystals. The identity of the calcium phosphate deposits in soft tissues as apatite has been proved by Taylor and Sheard (1929). Roseberry *et al.* (1931) and Yu and Blumenthal (1963) who have compared X-ray diffraction patterns of bone,

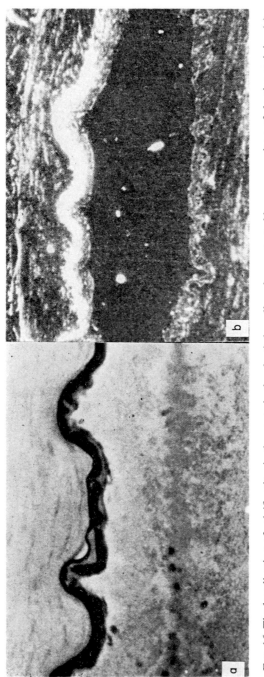

FIG. 16. The localisation of calcification in the aorta in the elastic lamellae, demonstrated by a comparison of elastica staining (a) and microincineration (b) of serial sections of human aorta. ($\times 350$)

teeth, various calcified soft tissue and isolated aortic elastic fibres with podolite ($Ca_3(PO_4)_2CaCO_3$) and hydroxy apatite ($3.Ca_3(PO_4)_2.Ca(OH)_2$) and demonstrated the identity of structure.

The dermis

General structure. The skin consists of two major layers of tissue with various appendages attached to the underlying organs by a loose subcutaneous faschia. The outermost layer, the epidermis, consists of stratified squamous epithelial cells varying in thickness from site-to-site on the body, and except in as far as it covers and protects the inner layer of the dermis and is attached to it by means of cellular processes which protrude from the lower surface, having no direct relationship with the connective tissues as a whole. In addition to the keratogenic cells of the epidermis, this region also contains melanotic granules which determine the overall colour of the skin. The epidermis develops from the ectoderm, but the inner layer, the corium, arises from the parietal mesoderm in common with other species of connective tissue, differentiating from the loose subcutaneous tissue during foetal growth. Penetrating the dermis to varying depths are hair follicles, and sweat and sebaceous glands. They develop as outgrowths of the lower layer, the *stratum germinativum*, of the epidermis into the corium, and again, except for the fact that the corium cells differentiate to form the outer hair root sheath and the walls of the sebaceous gland, they are not specifically associated with the connective tissue of the dermis. From the larger blood vessels in the loose subcutaneous tissue a network of smaller vessels penetrates the lower levels of the corium terminating in capillary beds which supply and drain the sweat glands, fat deposits, sebaceous glands and hair follicles. These vessels are similar in structure to others elsewhere in the body containing either elastic lamellae, collagen and smooth muscle or mainly collagen and smooth muscle depending on their size. They may, therefore, also be classed as connective tissue elements, but except in specialised tissues which have a rich capillary supply, represent only a minor component of the corium, especially in the upper immediately sub-epidermal portion of this section of the skin. The papillary regions of the skin are also served by a system of lymph capillaries which drain into larger components of the lymphatic system is the subcutaneous tissue. Certain specialised tissues such as the penis, the scrotum, the nipple and the perineum which can change their shape and size in response to external or internal stimuli contain considerable numbers of smooth muscle fibres over and above those associated with the blood vessels and this is also true of hirsute areas of the body, where *erector pili* muscles are present in association with each group of hair follicles to raise the hairs in response to stimuli. With the exception of the efferent nerves supplying these areas rich in smooth muscle, the majority of dermal nerve endings are sensory.

The dermis consists of collagen bundles which are loosely arranged in a rhomboid network with individual bundles lying at angles to one another. Intertwined amongst the collagen bundles lie single elastic fibres. Sections cut at right angles to the epidermal surface and stained for elastin demonstrate the apparently haphazard alignment of the elastica-staining elements in planes parallel with the surface at all levels beneath the dermal-epidermal junction. This layer which divides the dermis from the superficial epidermis, stains with elastica stains, and appears to be a continuous sheet irrespective of the direction of sectioning. The network of collagen bundles although composed of inextensible fibres (p. 27) is itself extensible as the bundles rotate relative to one another to form parallel alignments. Although it cannot be proved directly either by light or electron microscopy, it would appear likely that the return of the network to its unstretched orientation is brought about by the interwoven elastic fibres, much in the same way that a network composed of crossed rigid rods held together by elastic bands (Fig. 17) will return to its original shape when the forces exerted on diagonally opposed corners are removed.

Throughout the body the skin exhibits varying degrees of tension (Dupuytren, 1834; Langer, 1861; Cox, 1941) which may be ascribed to alterations in the "weave" of the elastin fibres among the collagen bundles.

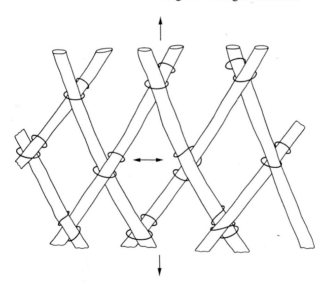

FIG. 17. Diagrammatic representation of the possible involvement of elastin fibres in the maintenance of the structure and tone of the skin network. The network of collagen bundles can be distorted by the application of a force in one direction, but returns to its original form when the force is removed, in exactly the same fashion that a network of rigid rods will resume its shape if each crossing point is restricted by an elastic band.

All these components of the skin may suffer change with age, ranging from loss of hair due to the atrophy of the hair follicle, to loss of tone, laxity and wrinkling of the skin as a whole. These will be dealt with in detail in so far as they are dependent on changes in the connective tissue elements in the dermis as a whole.

Morphology of ageing skin. Many workers have made histological studies on ageing skin, typical of which are the recent observations of Boisson *et al.* (1973) who have reported changes in skin using the light and the electron microscope. They stained samples of skin from the outer aspect of the upper arm with a variety of stains to reveal both elastin and collagen, and after osmic acid fixation cut thin sections for the electron microscope. They divided the ageing skins which they stained into four groups depending on the distribution of elastin fibres and collagen fibre bundles. Type O is indistinguishable from normal, having many elastic fibres running parallel to the epidermis in the deep sub-papillary region. The collagen bundles are closely packed and well organised, and especially in the deeper layers the dermis is essentially devoid of elastin fibres, the few that do exist being poorly stained. Types II and III represent a progressive reduction in elastin fibre number, and a fragmentation and disorientation of the collagen bundles. Even when the most pronounced alterations are apparent, the deep layers retain their elastin and the collagen still appears undegraded.

Senile purpura. The skin of the elderly is characteristically wrinkled and thin, especially in exposed sites such as the backs of the hands, the outer aspects of the forearms, the face and the neck. In these regions the skin shows an obvious loss of elasticity often hanging in folds, especially over regions in which it has been subjected to continuous extension and relaxation cycles throughout life such as over the elbows and along the angle of the jaw. Relatively slight trauma can result in intradermal extravasation of blood due to rupture of one or more of the capillaries. These purplish-brown spots which are often seen on the skin of elderly subjects have given rise to the term *senile purpura* to describe the condition (Tattersall and Savile, 1950). The incidence of senile purpura rises from 25% at 60 years of age to over 70% in the 9th decade.

The occurrence of purpura is directly associated with loose and thinning skin, and it might be assumed that one cause of capillary disruption might be the lack of tone in the dermis resulting in greater mobility of the small vessels which are normally protected by the firm dermis through which they pass. It is therefore, very much of a paradox that these regions contain high concentrations of elastica-staining material, the very substance which by virtue of its elastic properties might be expected to protect the capillaries against accidental trauma (Kissmeyer and With, 1922; Dick, 1947; Tattersall and Savile, 1950). Kissmeyer and With pointed out that these changes start to be apparent relatively early in life (i.e. well before subjects manifest signs of purpura) but they also observed most marked changes in exposed sites from fair-haired individuals. This was confirmed by Dick (1947) and Tattersall and Savile (1950), and although Ejiri (1936, 1937) did not differentiate between exposed and covered skin surfaces, his general observations were in close agreement with the negative findings of Hill and Montgomery (1940) who could report no changes in skin from covered sites of the body. In general there appears to be an increase in elastica-staining material in the exposed skin tissue of elderly subjects at the expense of collagen-staining fibres (Fig. 18). Slater (1966) made a detailed study of the reaction of senile dermis to the various elastica stains. Although certain dyes stain elastic tissue fairly selectively, their absolute specificity has been in doubt. Fullmer and Lillie (1957) have shown that variations in the degree of blockage of reactive groups on the surface of the collagen fibre can render it susceptible to staining with the resorcinol-fuchsin group of stains, and Hall and Saxl (1961) using Hart's modification of Weigert's stain were able to show that certain degraded collagens could be stained as elastin, in agreement with the very much earlier observations of Unna (1896) who divided the components of old or pathological connective tissue into collagen, collastin, collacin, elacin and elastin, depending on their degree of affinity for collagen and/or elastica stains. Gillman *et al.* (1955a, b) have developed stains with the express purpose of differentiating between connective tissue components which are related both to collagen and elastin. These stains have, however, not been applied widely to changes in the senile dermis.

Slater observed that both the collagenous and elastic elements of dermis suffer changes due to age and exposure, but that the rates at which these alterations in their staining properties take place may vary from site to site. There may, for instance, appear to be an increase in the number of elastic fibres in certain sites due to the collagen being degraded more rapidly than the elastin, thus providing a situation in which an increased proportion of the fibrous components of the dermis take up elastica stains. Elastic tissue also may undergo degenerative changes as can be shown by its increasing uptake of Alcian Blue and metachromatic dyes, indicating that glycosaminoglycans which are closely bound within the fibres in early life become more loosely attached and stainable with increasing age. The elastic fibres also lose their affinity for stains such as Mallory's phosphotungstic acid haematoxylin and Mason's Trichrome stain. At an even later stage in degeneration the elastic fibres appear as large swollen whorled fibres which may be surrounded by granular amorphous masses which still stain as elastin.

From these various observations and those of Boisson *et al.* (1973), it appears likely that age changes occur in both the collagen and the elastin

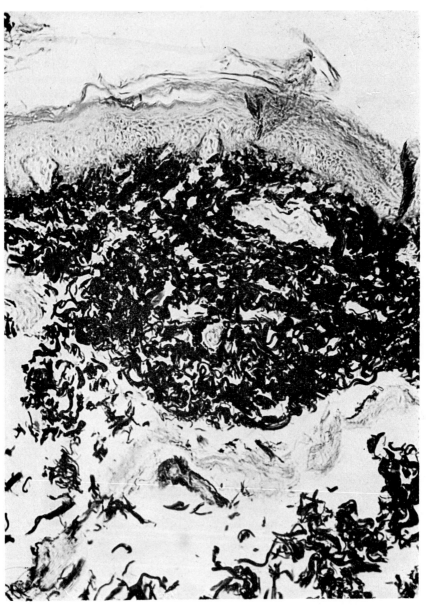

FIG. 18. Section of skin from the outer aspect of the forearm of an 82-year old woman stained with Weigart's elastica stain. ($\times$250)

components of dermis with increasing age, but that such changes can be accentuated by the simultaneous effects of exposure. In many instances the changes in aged covered skin are very slight (types O and I of Boisson's classification) and this has led a number of workers to claim that all the changes in the exposed sites are due to the action of ultra-violet irradiation alone (Sams and Smith, 1961; Smith *et al.*, (1962a, b, c). Smith *et al.* state that the profound alterations which occur in skin which has been subjected to prolonged exposure to active radiations are quite different from those occurring in aged skin, but since their claims are based equally on biochemical observations on ageing and irradiated skin, discussion of this will be left until the biochemical observations are considered (p. 106).

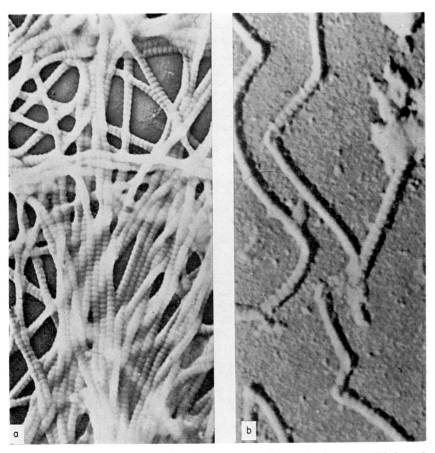

FIG. 19. Electron microscope studies of young covered (a) and old, exposed (b) dermal collagen. (a) ×15 000; (b) ×60 000)

Dawber and Shuster (1971) have examined sections of normal and irradiated skin in the scanning electron microscope and have reported a loss of
organised collagen bundles and the superimposition on the mat of disorganised
collagen fibres of a massive branching network, which appears to merge into
the larger masses of tissue. This observation is in close agreement with the
findings of Tunbridge et al. (1952) who, using the less sophisticated methods
of electron microscopy then available, demonstrated that those areas which
contained masses of elastica-staining material in the subepidermal region of
exposed skin, centained broken and bent collagen fibres coated with an
amorphous mass (Fig. 19). Tunbridge et al. (1952) also demonstrated that
the partial degradation of collagen with pepsin not only altered its structure,
so that it resembled the amorphous material mentioned above, but also
rendered it susceptible to staining with elastica stains.

Keech and Reed (1957) demonstrated that any effect which could be attributed to ultra-violet radiation was restricted to the *in vivo* situation. The
prolonged irradiation of pieces of post mortem skin tissue did not affect its
staining properties or electron microscopic appearance at all.

Load extension relationships of skin. The tensile strength of skin, i.e. the
force required to rupture it, has been determined *in vitro* by Rollhauser (1950)
and Yamada (1970). Rollhauser stated that the tensile strength increased
from 0.25–0.3 kg/mm² at 3 months of age to 2.05 kg/mm² in a 50–80 year
old age group. Yamada showed that the value rose from 0.4 to 2.6 kg/mm²
over a similar range of ages, and determined the extension at rupture which
also changes with age.

In vivo, skin extends two-dimensionally, either by the distension of the rib
cage during inhalation, flexure of the knee, elbow or knuckle joints, or
"experimentally" when a piece of skin is pinched between thumb and fore-
finger, and raised from the underlying tissue. Dick (1951) studied two-
dimensional distension *in vitro* by exerting hydrostatic pressure on a diaphragm composed of a circular piece of skin mounted over a piston. The
deflection of the centre of the diaphragm was amplified by a lever, and the
displacement measured. Grahame and Holt (1969) developed this method for
use *in vivo*, raising a circular piece of skin by the application of reduced pressure and calculating the height of the centre of the piece of tissue displaced.
They adapted the formula derived by Tregear (1966)

$$\text{Stress} = \frac{pa^2\left(1+\frac{x^2}{a}2\right)}{4\times d} \text{Strain}$$

where p = pressure, a = radius of diaphragm, x = height of the domed
distortion of the diaphragm, and d = thickness of skin, to calculate stress/
strain relationships from the measurements they were able to make. By

introducing the appropriate relationship between strain, pressure and the thickness of the skin, this equation can be converted into one which depends solely on the radius and height of the dome.

$$\text{Stress} = \frac{2x^2}{3a^2\left(1+\dfrac{2x^2}{a^2}\right)}$$

The top of the chamber through which the negative pressure is applied is connected to precision-bore tubing, and the volume of the dome of the skin, and hence the dimensions a and x are calculated from measurements of the column of liquid in the tube when the negative pressure is applied. Skin thickness can be measured by the use of Harpenden Calipers (Tanner and Whitehouse, 1955) using the skin fold above the dorsum of the hand over the fourth metacarpal bone, an area stated by McConkey et al. (1963) to be virtually free of subcutaneous fat. From data obtained in this fashion, Grahame and Holt (1969) calculated Young's Moduli for male and female subjects ranging in age from 19 to 83 years. The values for females rose by 1×108 dyne/cm^2/decade whereas those for male skin rose by 3×107 dyne/cm^2/decade. The absolute values which in youth range from 1.0×10^8 to 10×10^8 were of similar order to those recorded by other workers using in vitro extension and close to the level for purified collagen fibres (Buck, 1954). Grahame and Holt's method was based on the assumption that the skin not only obeyed Hooke's Law at any one age, but continued to do so at all ages. They claimed that this was true at extensions over 5%. They also made the tacit assumption that the dome which was elevated under reduced pressure was a segment of a sphere, and hence that the skin distended equally in any pair of mutually perpendicular planes at right angles to its surface. This latter assumption is not, however, true. Dupuytren (1834) and Langer (1861) observed that circular punctate incisions through the skin, resulted in the development of lenticular wounds, and Cox (1941) was able to deduce that the tension in the skin was greater in certain directions than in others at right angles. On the basis of these observations he was able to plot a series of lines on the surface of the body along which the skin tension was greatest – the so-called Langer's Lines. Ridge and Wright (1965a, b) have demonstrated that the physical properties of the skin parallel to these lines differ from those measured at right angles to them. Hence the raised dome would be a segment of an ovoid body rather than a segment of a sphere, and calculated values for its height would be incorrect. Ridge and Wright (1966a, b) demonstrated that the load extension curve was not linear as would be expected if Hooke's Law were to be obeyed (Fig. 20). Even the central portion of the curve (Phase B), although approaching linearity, does not uphold the assumptions of Grahame and Holt (1969) that linearity supervenes after 5% extension has been passed.

The three phases of the curve can be ascribed to totally different aspects of the extension cycle. Phase A, in which little load is required to accomplish a considerable degree of extension, may be due to the alignment of collagen bundles. In the relaxed skin, collagen bundles lie at an angle to one another, and their rotation relative to one another permits the tissue to be extended in

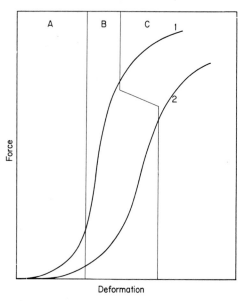

FIG. 20. Load/extension curves of two samples of skin: (1) 85 years of age, (s) 17 years of age. The portion of the curve B is the one for which the equation $E = c + kL^b$ has been proposed by Ridge and Wright (1965a).

the direction of the applied force without any stress being transmitted to the individual collagen bundles themselves. The relatively small proportion of elastic tissue which is present in skin (Varadi and Hall, 1965), may also be extended during this phase of extension of the whole tissue, and it may be that it is the long range elasticity of this component (see below) which returns the network of collagen bundles to its non-aligned state when the load is removed (Hall, 1976b). This straightening out process can be observed under the microscope (Craik and McNeil, 1966) and Ridge and Wright (1965a, b) have shown that the shape of this portion of the load/extension curve can be expressed by the equation:

$$E = xy \log L$$

Where E is the extension, L the load and x and y are constants which are dependent on the size of the tissue sample used for testing and the dimensions of the apparatus.

The central portion of the curve (Phase B) represents that section in the extension cycle in which the already aligned collagen bundles are themselves subjected to extension. There is no sharp discontinuity between phases A and B, some bundles being fully aligned before others, and the choice of the position of the vertical line dividing the two phases is completely arbitrary, merely indicating that at this point the majority of the collagen bundles are aligned whereas few are stretched. According to Ridge and Wright (1965a, b) this central portion of the load/extension curve can be characterised by the empirical equation:

$$E = c = kL^b$$

in which E and L again refer to extension and load, and c, k and b are constants. c and k are dependent on the size and shape of the test piece, k being related to the number of collagen fibres being stretched and to the orientation of the test piece relative to Langer's Lines. b on the other hand is completely independent of the dimension of either tissue or apparatus, and appears to represent alterations in the nature of the collagen fibres themselves. That this equation reflects the extension of a fully oriented skin collagen network, is adequately demonstrated by the observations of Ridge and Wright (1965a, b) on rat tail tendon for which the load/extension curve can also be described by a simple power relationship, of exactly similar form to that which is applicable to skin.

The third phase of the extension curve represents the situation in which rupture of individual fibres builds up until final cleavage of the specimen occurs.

The shapes of load/extension curves of young and old skins are similar (Fig. 20), but they differ in the amount of extension induced by any given load. The relationship, between this variation in extension and the age of the subject, is a complex one, but Ridge and Wright (1966a) have shown that there is an important relationship between values for the exponential factor "b" and the age of the individual subject (Fig. 21). Values for "b" rise with increasing age over the age range 0 to 45 years for both males and females, falling again at ages between 50 and 80 years. Hall (1967) has commented that rising values of "b" indicate an increasing "stiffness" of the fibres, whereas the subsequent reduction in value can only imply that a "loosening" of the structure takes place with increasing age. Cross-linkages may explain the increasing values observed during the first 40 years of life, but it is unlikely that cross-linkages once formed will subsequently be broken. One must, therefore, look for some other explanation of this falling off with age, such as the fission of peptide linkages in the main protein chains. This possibility is dealt with in more detail in the section on pseudoelastins. Hall (1967) has suggested that the peak values of "b" in the region of 40–50 years of age may be regarded as representing a period of minimum entropy. Before that time the tissue proteins are becoming more firmly attached to one another, and the individual chains are becoming more markedly oriented. After the peak period the fission of main chains renders the whole collagen structure less organised and more easily extensible.

It may be assumed that the two phenomena, maturation and senescence, proceed simultaneously and that at the point of minimum entropy the senescent process supersedes the maturation one.

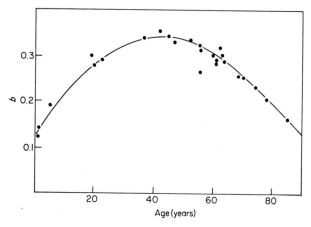

FIG. 21. Changes in the exponential coefficient "b" in the equation $E = c + kL^b$ which describes the middle portion of the load/extension curve for skin (male) (after Ridge and Wright, 1965a).

Other equations varying slightly from that of Ridge and Wright, have been proposed by Glaser *et al.* (1965); Kennedi *et al.* (1965) and Elden (1970). In all of them the relationship of E and L in the second phase of the load/extension curve is expressed in a more or less complicated power form. Only Ridge and Wright (1964, 1965a, b, 1966a, b) report stiffening followed by loosening, probably due to the fact that the majority of the other studies have been carried out on rat or rabbit skin, usually from birth to maturity, and thus do not reflect any ageing effect at all. Reports on age changes in the "toe" part of the curve are somewhat conflicting. Some workers have observed the toe to be less steep with increasing age (Dick, 1951) others suggest that it disappears completely (Kennedi *et al.*, 1965) while Jansen and Rottier (1957) did not observe any variation in the shape of the toe at all. This may be due in part to the fact that it is very difficult to determine the exact point at which the load starts to be applied, without subjecting the specimen to simultaneous observation under a microscope (Viidik, 1972, 1973). As mentioned earlier

the elastin content of the skin may determine the shape of the toe, and variations in elastin content (Dick, 1951; Slater and Hall, 1973) may affect this
early stage of the extension cycle (Daly, 1969).

Viidik (1973) has studied the physical performance of skin as a function of
time and has developed more complex analyses of the relationship between
stress and strain than those derived by other workers such as Ridge and
Wright. He showed that the value for the stiffness factor which would, in a
linear extension curve be termed the Young's Modulus, is not independent of
time, rates of application of load being of importance in determining how
skin stretches under load. Little is known about the way the visco-elasticity
and plasticity of skin changes with age. Rollhauser (1950) reported that con-
secutive stress-strain curves shifted to the right in tissues from new-born
animals, whereas the changes which were apparent in the stress-strain curves
of mature animals were mostly confined to the toe phase; the average slope,
curvature and position of the higher regions of the curves being less affected
by subsequent extension cycles.

The skeleton

The supporting tissues of the body consist of the calcified bony components,
and the interosseous cartilage organised into a sophisticated weight bearing
framework. Each tissue entity differs from the others in composition, the only
major fibrous component which is common to bone, cartilage and intervertebral disc being collagen. Because of this continuity it is possible to con-
sider the ageing of the skeleton as a whole, even though the individual regions
may be subjected to differing ageing processes.

Bone. Bone is formed by the deposition of calcium salts onto an organic
matrix which itself constitutes between 30% and 40% of the dry material in
the bone. By far the largest proportion of the matrix consists of collagen
(between 90% and 95%), and whereas the collagen of the soft tissues is in the
main relatively resistant to turn over (see p. 151), the whole of the bone mass,
both matrix and mineral, is capable of undergoing continuous dynamic trans-
formation. Looked at as an entire tissue, bone suffers continual resorption
and under normal circumstances the mass of tissue lost by resorption is
replaced by a concomitant degree of resynthesis. Since this degree of replacement occurs continuously, few if any individual elements of the bony structure
are retained long enough to demonstrate ageing phenomena *per se*. Any ageing effects which can be observed in the skeleton as a whole, and which are
attributable to changes in the bone, must therefore, be due to an imbalance
of anabolic and catabolic activities.

Osteoporosis. It has long been appreciated that relatively massive bone loss
occurs with advancing age. This manifests itself in the human subject most

markedly in a loss of height. Dent and Watson (1966) have shown for instance, that "normally" ageing subjects may lose as much as 5 cm in total height within relatively short periods of time (1 to 3 years) especially in the case of women at the menopause. Few studies have been made of total height loss for individuals over the whole period from around 30 years of age, when full maturity may be assumed to have been attained, to 80–90 years of age when the degenerative changes may well have reached a maximum. There is, however, ample evidence that the overall height loss may be as great as 8 cm over this period. In one longitudinal study, Miall et al. (1967) have reported on four surveys in Wales and have shown that the mean reduction in height over the period 40 to 70 is between 1.25 and 2.0 cm/decade irrespective of sex. In their studies there does not appear to be any accelerated height loss due to the menopause, and since they follow the same cohorts throughout, this failure to observe a menopausal effect cannot be ascribed to the ironing out of a series of individual height reductions due to variations in the age at which menopause occurs. As opposed to these observations, Henneman and Wallach (1957) had observed that oestrogen therapy which might be expected to repair the hormonal imbalance occasioned by the menopause, prevented further height loss immediately after the commencement of treatment in 69% of females; even in those who had suffered a height loss of up to 3.5 cm per decade. Of the remainder all but 1% stabilised at only slightly below the height at which they started treatment, within one or two years. The question of the hormonal control of bone loss is, therefore, not yet fully answered, but it must be borne in mind that part of the reduction in stature might be due to changes in the intervertebral discs in which appreciable morphological changes occur, especially in cases of pronounced spinal osteoporosis.

Osteoporotic changes can occur in all the bony structures of the body, in both cancellous and trabelular regions of bone, but are normally confined to the spine, pelvis, and more rarely, the skull and the extremities. This statement is based on that definition of the condition which is subscribed to by most pathologists and in the past by radiologists as well. To the pathologist the term osteoporosis means that the amount of histochemically identifiable bone is diminished relative to the total area of a histological section, and by extrapolation that the mass of bone per unit volume is decreased. This may, therefore, be referred to as a reduction in bone density. Unfortunately, the same term – bone density – has been employed by radiologists to indicate the degree of translucency of a radiograph, particularly of the vertebrae. An increased translucency can be associated with a loss of mineralised tissue, and this manifests itself as a decreased density in the radiograph, but such a loss of radioopacity need not necessarily be due to the type of overall bone loss which is defined as osteoporosis. It could be occasioned by decalcification such as occurs in osteomalacia. It has been demonstrated that in cases of frank osteoporosis, the density of a spinal radiograph, obtained under standardised conditions, and compared with the density of a radiograph of an aluminium wedge, can be correlated directly with the weight of ash derived from unit volume of bone removed at autopsy (Fig. 22). The degree of standardisation

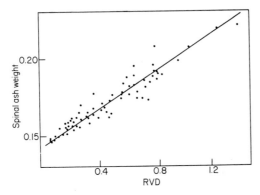

FIG. 22. The relationship between "spinal ash weight" – the weight of ash in unit volume of incinerated vertebra and "RVD" – an arbitrary parameter relating to the density of a standard X-ray picture of the same region.

and correction for soft tissue effects which have to be made to permit the quantitative assessment of osteoporosis from such spinal X-rays is, however, quite considerable, and alternative methods of *in vivo* assessment have been devised. Nordin and Horsman (1970), Exton-Smith (1973) and Dequeker *et al.* (1971) have shown that an assessment of osteoporosis which is in all ways comparable to that derived from spinal radiology, can be obtained by measurements of the cortical thickness of the metacarpal bone. Since at its mid length this bone is essentially cylindrical, measurement of the overall diameter D and the internal diameter of the cortex d can provide a measurement which is directly related to the area of the cortical annulus (Fig. 23). If this is then described as a proportion of the total area of the cross-section of the bone by

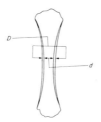

FIG. 23. The method for the calculation of the "metacarpal index". The inner and outer diameters of the cortical cylinder are measured on hand X-rays, and the index calculated from D^2-d^2/D as a percentage.

dividing the overall diameter D, a figure is obtained which, expressed as a percentage, is known as the metacarpal index. The changes of this index with age (Fig. 24) and disease are directly comparable with the more difficultly determinable spinal parameters. Morgan and Newton-John (1969) have shown that using this type of approach the amount of bone lost can be shown to amount to about 40% of the optimum bone mass.

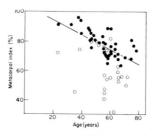

FIG. 24. The relationship between metacarpal index and age for two groups of female subjects. ●, normal subjects; ○, rheumatoid arthritic subjects treated with prednisolone.

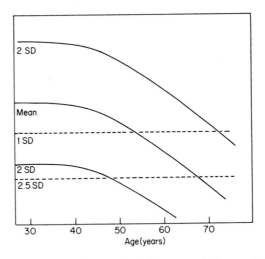

FIG. 25. Model curve for bone loss (after Morgan and Newton-John, 1969). The upper and lower solid lines represent a distribution 2 standard deviations above and below the mean value. The dotted lines represent 1 and 2.5 standard deviations below the mean value at age 30. These indicate that by 70 years of age an appreciable proportion of the upper segment of the normal distribution has lost bone to an extent which brings it below the majority of the values at maturity.

They were able to show that there is a Gaussian distribution of the values for the amounts of bone measurable at each age. It is, therefore, justifiable to plot mean curves for the rate of bone loss for the population with parallel lines one standard deviation above and below to cover the spread. A model curve with these characteristics is shown in Fig. 25. When real figures from the observations of Odland *et al.* (1958), Nordin *et al.* (1965) and Nordin (1966) are plotted in this way, it can be seen that the average amounts of bone diminish with age, but that the loss begins between 15 and 25 years earlier in women than in men. The amounts of bone vary considerably at any one age, the standard deviation being about 12% of the mean value. Morgan and Newton-John (1969) point out that when taken together with the 40% reduction in total bone mass, which can occur in the case of female subjects between 40 and 80 years of age, this marked variability means that one woman in 200 will only have the same amount of bone at 35 as the average woman has at 75. Males, as well as starting to lose bone at a later age, lose it more slowly than women. The two rates of bone loss remain roughly constant with age at about 5% per decade for men and 10% per decade for women. Thus allowing for the fact that in general men have a more robust skeleton at maturity than women, the level of calcified tissue remaining in the eighth and ninth decades is appreciably less in women than in men. If it is assumed that a certain bone density is required to resist the effects of traumatic insults such as slight falls, this differential between male and female bone loss may account for the different incidence of fractures in the two sexes.

Jowsey (1960) has shown that the pattern of bone turnover changes with increasing age. The resorption of bone tissue increases with age, whereas, the formation of bone remains at a relatively constant level. Resorption occurs at the bone surface, and there is little difference between the surface activity of either cortical or trabecular tissue. The surface area of the latter, however, because of its much looser structure, is approximately three times greater than that of the cortex, and hence when expressed in terms of unit bone volume the rate of loss of the trabecular region is far more dramatic than the decrease in cortical regions (Figs 26a and b).

At a morphological level bone turnover can be assessed mainly by histochemical techniques. The presence of uncalcified osteoid is recognised as being associated with areas of bone formation, whilst the existence of lacunae indicates previous or current resorption (Frost and Villaneuva, 1960).

The mean amounts of bone present in a specific portion of the skeleton, together with the appropriate standard deviation to define the scatter, may be taken as representing the "physiological" osteoporosis typical of the age group concerned. There are, however, especially in the upper age groups, individuals who have clinically identifiable symptoms which indicate that their degree of osteoporosis is appreciably greater than should be expected from subjects of their age. These subjects usually present in hospital with marked back pain, often with a high degree of spinal curvature, and at X-ray,

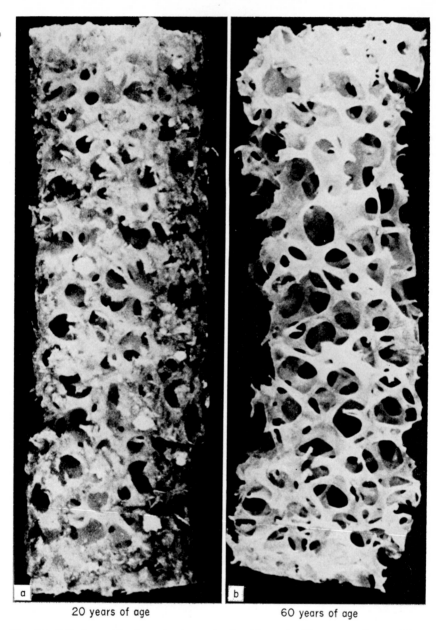

20 years of age   60 years of age

FIG. 26. Cylinders of fat-free, dry bone obtained from the iliac crests of two subjects age (a) 20 years of age, and (b) 60 years of age, showing the normal degree of bone loss associated with age. ($\times 12$) (Reproduced with the permission of Dr. J. Dequeker.)

they are seen to have vertebral bodies with collapsed or distorted end plates, and often have numerous microfractures of the spinal processes. Quantitatively these subjects show a level of bone density which is considerably lower than is typical of their age group and as will be shown later (p. 169) demonstrate marked alterations in the amount and nature of the collagen component of a variety of other connective tissues throughout the body. Little is known of the aetiology of this "pathological" degree of osteoporosis, but similar changes can result from Cushing's Syndrome (Jowsey, 1966) or from treatment with artificial corticosteroids (Hall, 1976a). Nordin et al. (1972) have shown that in the elderly, osteoporosis is often accompanied by osteomalacia due to diets deficient in calcium and/or vitamin D, and to lack of sunlight (either because the elderly subjects are house-bound or through choice) necessary for the conversion of ergosterol and 7-dehydrocholesterol to vitamins D_2 and D_3.

Loss of mineral material from the bone also affects the apparent bone density, but since it does so without having any effect on the bone matrix it should perhaps not be regarded as a true connective tissue effect. Methods other than X-ray densitrometry are required to assess the connective tissue changes. These will be considered in the section dealing with chemical and biochemical changes associated with ageing.

Articular cartilage. The function of articular cartilage is to facilitate the movement of one bone surface over another, while bearing a load, which even during a relatively non-energetic activity such as walking, may amount to between four and five times body weight (Dowson et al., 1968). Any deviations from its ideal structure due to ageing or disease, may be expected to result in impaired joint action. A massive degree of joint degeneration occurs in cases of rheumatoid arthritis, but as yet the cause of this pathological condition is not fully understood. A variety of suggestions have been considered to explain the changes which are observed, ranging from microbiological infection through the immunological activation of tissues to attack by lysosomal enzymes to localised degradation due to trauma.

Although some if not all of these factors may have a role to play in the massive destruction of joint surfaces which can be observed in advanced states of arthritis, one or other of the endogenous ones might be of universal significance, and could be the direct result of the ageing process. Looked at from another point of view it is in fact quite remarkable that many joints are able to tolerate, for periods of from 70 to 80 years, repeated loading to levels which, for instance when the subject lands from a relatively small jump, may amount to between 250 and 300 kg. In the case of the knee joint a low degree of geometrical congruity means that these loads may be carried on an area of cartilage measuring less than 5 cm². Loading, is however, seldom static, being a complex mixture of sliding, rolling and direct percussion phenomena. Similarly the effect of loading is distributed not only over the bearing surface of the cartilage, but also among the ligaments, the synovial membrane and through the attached tendons to the peri-articular muscles, and this must protect the joint to a certain extent. Even so an appreciable amount of the repetitive impact must be absorbed by the cartilage, and it is its structure which helps to protect the joint and provides it with the degree of resilience required for normal function.

The actual load bearing surface of the synovial joint consists of a layer of specialised connective tissue about 1–7 mm thick in healthy young joints, less in osteoarthosic joints. This hyaline layer contains a densely packed three-dimensional network of collagen fibrils 20–30 nm in diameter demonstrating the 64 nm cross striations typical of normal collagen. The bundles lie roughly parallel to the articular surface, and are interspersed with ground substance and with lenticular cells which are also aligned, parallel to the surface. Deeper layers contain a more random alignment of collagen fibres, and the cells assume a more spherical outline. With increasing age the deeper layers become oriented more nearly at right angles to the bearing surface (Barnett *et al.*, 1961).

The upper layers of the cartilage contain 70% water, about one third of which is located within the cells. The remainder is bound to the glycosamino-glycans of the ground substance. Some at least of this may be expressed from the cartilage during loading to form a lubrication film between the opposing joint surfaces.

The continued mechanical stresses to which the joint is subjected through-out life may result in the attrition and removal of the finer collagen fibrils from the surface, revealing the coarser underlying bundles. Certainly super-ficial surveys of the cartilage surface by engineering techniques demonstrate slight increases in surface roughness with increasing age. (Wright *et al.*, 1973) (Fig. 27), although these changes are in no sense as great as those which are

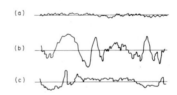

FIG. 27. Talysurf recordings of surface irregularities of human cartilage. (a) Femoral condyle, age 26; (b) Osteoarthrosic femoral condyle, age 63; (c) Femoral head, age 67. The vertical scale is 1000×actual rugosities; the horizontal scale is 100× actual length of specimen.

associated with osteoarthrosis. The amount of fluid retained within the carti-lage, and available for lubrication purposes is dependent on the nature of the glycosaminoglycans. These change markedly with increasing age (cf. p. 136), and the water content will alter accordingly.

The intervertebral disc. Between each pair of vertebrae lies a disc of material consisting in youth of an elastic wall – the annulus fibrosus – enclosing a gel-like central portion – the nucleus pulposus. In this state the disc fulfils its function as a shock absorber distributing vertical force or shock outwards where it is taken up by the peripheral ligaments. Pressure exerted through the vertebral end plates onto the central gel-like structure of the nucleus is dispersed and transformed into radial forces which tend to expand the annulus. The fibrillar structure of the annulus is such that the majority of the fibrils lie circumferentially around the nucleus and hence attempts to expand the annular ring result in linear forces along the length of each fibrillar ring (Fig. 28).

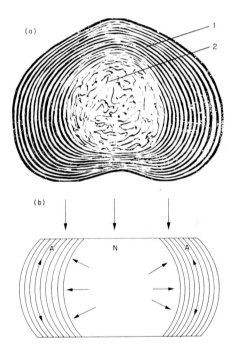

Fig. 28a. Diagram of transverse section through intervertebral disc. 1. Annulus fibrosus; 2. Nucleus pulposus. The appearance of randomly oriented fibrils in the latter indicate the age of the disc as above middle age.

Fig. 28b. Longitudinal section indicating how vertical compressive forces exerted on the end plate are transmitted radially through the nucleus (N) to distend the annulus (A) thus stretching the fibres in this region.

X-ray diffraction studies of freeze-dried annuli (Happey *et al.*, 1974) demon-strated that the "give" of the annulus, which is necessary for the disc as a whole to act as an ideal shock absorber, can occur even although the fibres themselves consist of inextensible collagen, since just as in the dermis they lie at an angle to the central plane of the disc. The expansion of the annulus under radial pressure from the compressed nucleus can therefore be seen to be brought about by a rotation of the fibres into the plane of the disc. Each circumferential layer of collagen fibres lies at roughly the same angle to the plane, but alternate layers are displaced on opposite sides of the plane.

With increasing age, random fibrosis of the disc occurs both in the annulus and in the nucleus. The super-position of randomly aligned fibres in amongst the highly crystalline regions of the annulus cannot markedly affect the physical properties of this portion of the disc, except in so far as the move-ment of the highly oriented collagen sheaths is restricted by the newly laid down mass of fibres.

In the nucleus on the other hand the replacement or infiltration of the gel-like structure of the youthful nucleus by a fibrous mat has a marked effect on the physical properties. Because the orientation of the fibres is random and totally three-dimensional the qualitative nature of the physical properties of the tissue is not changed, but quantitatively the elasticity and resilience of the nucleus is greatly decreased (Fig. 28; Hall *et al.*, 1976).

Happey *et al.* (1969) have reported on the X-ray diffraction analysis of the fibrous components of the elderly nucleus, and have shown that in addition to the collagen fibres, which after excision and alignment can be shown to have typical reflexions at 0.29 nm and 1.15 nm, a further component demonstrates little crystallinity but a defined reflexion at about 0.46 nm could also be identified. This has been studied by Blakey *et al.* (1962) and Little and Taylor (1964) and has been identified as a so-called β-protein. This component is identifiable in an increasing number of subjects over the age of 45 with a sharp increase from 11 to 71% in the percentage showing these typical X-ray findings between the age groups 31–45 and 46–60. All the sub-jects over 76 studied (Blakey *et al.*, 1962) showed evidence of β-protein.

β-Proteins are usually derived by the denaturation of soluble proteins. The latter which occur mixed with the glycosaminoglycans in the young nucleus may exist either in the random or α-coiled state, and it is possible that con-version of these to the insoluble denatured β-state may occur due to the repeated stresses which are exerted on the gel during the ageing process. During denaturation it is possible that the soluble proteins may become more firmly bound to the glycosaminoglycans with which they are surrounded. Hall (1970) has shown that this can occur *in vitro* in the case of soluble collagen which is stretched and relaxed repeatedly during precipitation. The resultant fibres are more resistant to solution in dilute acetic acid, and the acid-resistant fraction contains the greater proportion of the associated poly-saccharide. This may also explain to a certain extent the changes which can be observed in the water content of the nucleus with increasing age, since glycosaminoglycans bound to protein will have a lower moisture uptake than when in a free state.

The moisture content of the intervertebral disc has been studied by a number of workers (Püschel, 1930; Armstrong, 1965; Galante, 1967; Hall and Reed, 1973). All have shown that there is a progressive decrease in the amount of moisture present in the nucleus with increasing age. Expressing the moisture content as a function of the dry weight of tissue, Hall and Reed reported a fall from 4 to 2.8 in discs ranging from those of newly born male infants to those of 90-year old men, whereas comparable figures for female discs were 3.6 and 2.8. Both these sets of figures indicated a significant degree of dehydration ($p < 0.005$ and 0.05 respectively) which could go a long way towards explaining the lack of resilience observed in the nucleus with increasing age. The observations of Hall and Reed (1973) concerning the moisture content of the annulus were, however, not fully in agreement with those of Püschel (1930) who reported an age-mediated dehydration of this region of the disc as well. The relatively few subjects studied by Hall and Reed who were younger than 30 years of age did in fact show a trend towards dehydration, but from 40 to 90 years of age although there was a considerable scatter, the moisture content increased again by nearly 30% until at the end of life the moisture content of the disc was almost constant throughout the annulus and nucleus at between 2.0 and 3.0 times the weight of the dry tissue. In the same paper, Hall and Reed confirmed the fact that the majority of the fibrous material which appears in the nucleus with increasing age is non-collagenous in nature, the level of collagen in the nucleus rising by only 0.075% per year throughout life. However, above 65 years of age the proportion of collagen in the dry matter in the annulus increases by nearly 1% per year after remaining essentially constant before.

These changes in collagen content can be further demonstrated by a study of the compression characteristics of discs from various age groups. Hall *et al.* (1975) have devised an instrument in which compression under vertical load is measured in a cylinder of tissue, together with the lateral distortion in four mutually perpendicular directions, in a plane at right angles to the compression. From these various parameters, all the compressive moduli can be determined. The relationships between the values for these parameters, and the age and orientation of the tissue sample are complex, but certain factors can easily be demonstrated (Fig. 29). The distortion of the annulus which occurs preferentially in a radial sense, as the layers of collagen fibres are compressed does not change to any great extent with increasing age. The nucleus, however, which is more isotropic and is essentially gel-like and easily distorted by applied load, becomes more rigid with advancing age, and since the newly laid down fibres are arranged in a three-dimensional network, the four mutually perpendicular measurements of lateral distension are essentially equal.

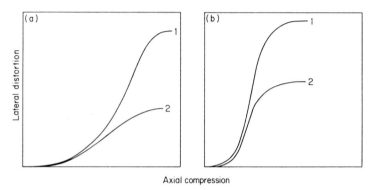

Axial compression

FIG. 29. The lateral distortion in two perpendicular planes induced by axial compression on cylinders of (a) annulus and (b) nucleus of human intevertebral discs.' In (a) curve 1 represents tracings for both young and old tissues in a radial direction, curve 2 along the axis of the circumferentially aligned fibres. In (b), where the tissue is isotropic, curve 1 represents the equal distortion in both perpendicular planes in young tissue, curve 2 the same effect in old tissue.

Connective tissues in the musculature

The tendons which anchor the musculature to the skeleton continue as collagenous sheaths around and between the muscle fibres. During ageing, the work capacity of individual muscles decreases. This may be due to a frank muscular dystrophy (Berg, 1956) or to changes in the muscle sheaths (Verzar, 1964). Schaub (1964) demonstrated that the amount of collagen in various muscles of the rat rose during the first few months of life, then remained constant until the twentieth month, when a rapid rise set in. In very old animals the collagen content amounts to almost double that in young adults. Verzar (1964) also recorded that the lability of the collagen, as measured by the technique of hydroxyproline estimation in the material taken into solution by heating for 10 min at 65 °C, is markedly reduced with age, falling from 40 % in 1–2-month old animals to 3–5 % by 30–40 months. From this it can be deduced that cross-link formation occurs increasingly with age in this type of connective tissue, just as in sites in which collagen occurs in more massive amounts. The increased rigidity of this connective tissue may well account for some of the dysfunction of the muscles which is apparent with increasing age.

Extracellular matrix of major organs

A similar phenomenon may account for the reduction with increasing age in the activity of certain of the major highly cellular organs of the body. The liver, for instance consists of a mass of cellular entities enmeshed in a connective tissue matrix. Since the products of the activity of one type of cell may require transportation to other cells for further metabolism, any factor which can change the penetrability of the intercellular matrix will alter the overall function of the organ, even although the individual cells may retain their activity unimpaired. An increase in the connective tissue component of the organ or a change in its properties could easily affect the permeability of the matrix. It has been demonstrated (Shock, 1964) that there is little evidence for cell loss in the liver with increasing age, and although there have been some reports of changes in the levels of individual enzymes (Barrows, 1956; Weinback and Garbus, 1956, 1959; Zorzoli, 1969) it would appear most likely that the presence of increasingly cross-linked collagen may account for an appreciable proportion of the organ dysfunction, by decreasing the permeability of the organ matrix.

The respiratory system

The lungs decrease in weight at advanced age. Howell (1970) quotes Reichenstein as indicating that on average there is a 21% reduction in the mass of both lungs between the ages of 60 and 90, although the actual weights of the two lungs remain different throughout life, the right lung being about 23% larger than the left. This loss of tissue is paralleled by a reduction in function. There is an impairment of gaseous exchange, and the arterial blood of an elderly subject has a lower oxygen saturation, equivalent in fact to that of a young adult breathing air from an altitude of between five and seven thousand feet.

Part at least of this loss of lung mass is due to a reduction in the thickness of the alveolar wall (Freeman, 1973). The loss of pulmonary function, however, is not associated with any increase in the alveolar basement membrane. The elastic fibres surrounding the ducts and the mouths of the alveoli are reduced in thickness and in number, but the overall elastic content of the lung increases with age, (Pierce and Ebert, 1965). The fraction of the pulmonary elastin which does increase has been shown to be localised in the pleural and septal tissues. There is no evidence for any disruption of the elastic fibres nor of their calcification. It must, therefore, be assumed that the changes in lung tissue are induced by different phenomena from those which affect the walls of the large blood vessels, where loss of elastic tissue, production of pseudoelastin and finally calcification occur progressively with ageing.

The eye

Changes in vision with age are well documented. Accommodation, namely the ability of the organism to alter the curvature of the lens to enable close objects to be focused on the retina, decreases with age. Starling (1941) records a variation in accommodation from 13.8 diopters in 10-year old human subjects to 1.1 diopters in 60-year old subjects. The rate at which accommmodation decreases is greatest over the age range 40 to 45 years, falling by 0.4 diopters a year over this period. This would appear to be due to progressive and relatively permanent changes in the morphology of the lens, which becomes set in the flat unaccommodated form in which it is able to resist the activity of the ciliary muscle, which in the young is capable of increasing the curvature of the anterior pole of the lens with a concomitant lengthening of the distance between the anterior and posterior surfaces and a reduction in the rear focal length of the lens as a whole. The major connective tissue component in this optical-mechanical element, is the lens capsule which not only contains the various proteins of the crystalline lens, but also acts as an elastic membrane determining the shape of the lens as a whole. The lens increases in size throughout life, because less tissue is being continuously laid down, without any concomitant removal of tissue. Smith (1883) was the first to demonstrate this and more recent studies have recorded a mean increase of lens thickness from 3.7 mm to 5.1 mm between 20 and 80 years of age (0.23 mm/ decade), (Leighton, 1973). The increase in size due to fibre deposition in the periphery of the lens is directly associated with increased rigidity, and hence longer focal length, leading to presbiopia or long-sightedness, and also because of a reduction in the transparency of the outer rim of the lens, of angle-closure glaucoma, in which the subject's peripheral vision is cut off. Kefalides (1969) and Spiro and Fukushi (1969) isolated a protein fraction from lens capsule with the typical amino acid analysis of collagen. These molecules were substituted on their hydroxyproline residues with glycans consisting of glucose and galactose. Other fractions containing sialic acid, fucose and glycosaminoglycans were also identified. In the normal eye the collagen molecules of the lens capsule are not capable of being formed into fibrils and it is probably the high concentration of polysaccharide which prevents this development from occurring.

In addition to its structural role the capsule may also have a metabolic role to play as can be shown by the presence of enzymes of the glycolytic pathway. It may have a positive function in the active transport of nutrients to the lens and in the interchange of ions and metabolites between the lens and the aqueous humour. The removal of collagen from the intact lens by incubation with collagenase, however, induced minimal changes in the active transport of ions in the lens (Becker and Collier, 1965) hence it may be assumed that the collagenous components of the lens capsule itself has little or no part to play in any metabolic function which may occur.

The vitreous, filling the body of the eye between the lens and the retina, although apparently structureless at low magnifications can be shown in the electron microscope to consist of a more dense cortical region surrounding a less dense central core (Schwarz, 1961). Balazs (1968) has commented on the value of the vitreous as a shock absorber, mitigating the disruptive effects of head movement on vision by maintaining the necessary distance between the rear surface of the lens and the retina. It is therefore, of interest that the morphology of the vitreous resembles that of the young intervertebral disc in consisting of a more fluid centre surrounded by a relatively rigid outer body. The outer layers of the vitreous consist of a fibrous mesh in which cells are embedded. These fibres have an amino acid analysis similar to that of collagen, but in the electron microscope do not show the 64 nm cross striations typical of mature collagen. They demonstrate a 12–25 nm periodicity similar to that which can be observed in foetal connective tissues from other sites (Schwarz, 1961; Fine and Tousimis, 1961). Again, as in the lens capsule, the almost complete transparency of the vitreous would appear to be due to the association of the collagen molecules with high concentrations of polysaccharide. Dische and Zelemenis (1955) isolated this polysaccharide, and showed that a major portion of it consists of a galactoglucan similar to that present in the lens capsule.

With increasing age the vitreous demonstrates clinical signs of deterioration, typified by the appearance of "floaters". These may be due to localised opacity of the vitreous humour itself, or may be the remains of structures remaining from the early development of the eye. They are not related in any way to the onset of cataract, which is a development occurring solely in the lens.

Cataract may occur as a generalised increase in opacity of the lens as a whole, or may be represented by a localised opacity, usually central, and known as nuclear sclerosis. Sippel (1965) has suggested that the reduction in the metabolic activity of the lens with increasing age which accompanies nuclear sclerosis may be due to a disproportionate increase in lens volume relative to surface area. Thus the central portion of the lens, being further from the capillary bed lying in the region of the ciliary muscles, is starved of nutrient material and the high molecular weight elements are no longer held in solution. It appears that this may be related to changes in the glutathione content of the lens, which is present in high concentration in the normal lens, but is greatly reduced in cataract.

3

Microstructural Changes in Connective Tissues with Age

The X-ray diffraction pattern

The diffraction of a beam of X-rays by the individual atoms of a molecule results in localised darkening of a photographic plate placed in the path of the reflected beam. Each darkened spot corresponds to a given atom of a reflexion plane, and it is possible to calculate inter atomic distances from spacings measured on the photographic plates. In the case of a molecule as complex as that of collagen only a limited number of orders of reflexion can be seen, the number of points at which the higher orders of reflexion can reinforce one another exactly, being very few (Fig. 30).

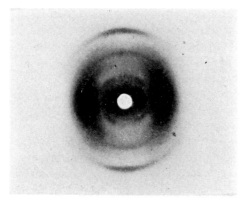

FIG. 30. X-ray diffraction diagram of fibrous collagen showing meridional and equatorial reflexions. The fact that the reflexions are arcs rather than discrete dots indicates the angle at which adjacent fibrils are aligned to the axis of the fibre.

Collagen

Early in the use of X-ray diffraction for the examination of the collagen molecule (Astbury, 1938; Astbury and Bell, 1940). it became apparent that one of the major meridional reflexions was due to some form of folding or coiling of the molecules. It was later calculated that the repeating distance

67

responsible for these spots in the diffraction pattern was one of 0.29 nm along the axis of the fibre and that this could represent the pitch of a helical coil. Cowan *et al.* (1955) showed that the small amount of stretching which collagen could withstand before rupture, resulted in this distance increasing to 0.31 nm. Many of the earlier structures suggested for collagen on the basis of this concept did not fit the X-ray diffraction pattern it was not appreciated at the time that it was unnecessary for there to be an integral number of residues in each turn of the helix. The observations of Pauling and Corey (1951); Crick (1954) and Ramachandran and Kartha (1955) concerning the possibility of non-integral numbers of residues between related regions of adjacent coils of the helix, paved the way for the evolution of the models of Rich and Crick (1955) and Ramachandran (1967) on which the presently accepted structure of collagen is based.

Individual points in the diffraction pattern of collagen are lengthened into arcs, indicating that the protein chains which have repeating structures every 0.3 nm, are aligned at different angles to the axis of the fibril. Similar angular displacement can be deduced from the longer molecular spacing (1.1 nm), associated with the less widely spaced series of equatorial reflections (Finean, 1967). Feitelberg and Kaunitz (1949) observed that the arcs were more intense when patterns from elderly subjects were studied, but that the displacement which could be calculated from the angle subtended at the centre of the diagram by the individual arcs was greatest during adolescence. Kratky *et al.* (1962) and Fels (1966) also observed a reduction in the spread of the arcs in later life, and from this it may be assumed that an increasing degree of parallel alignment occurs with advancing age.

Low angle X-ray diffraction also demonstrates an angular displacement about the axis, but in this case, the displacement has been shown to be due to the twisting together of the three individual monomeric collagen molecules to form the three-stranded super helix, tropocollagen. Treatment of collagen with hydrogen bond breaking reagents severs the linkages between the individual chains of young collagen which is without covalent cross-links, and the ordered structure associated with a well defined X-ray diffraction pattern is lost. Low angle patterns of collagen from older subjects still retain a well defined pattern even after treatment with guanidine hydrochloride, or other hydrogen bond breaking substances, due to the fact that the triple helical structure is stabilised by the introduction of co-valent cross-linkages during maturation (cf. p. 87).

The alignment of the molecules which is associated with increasing age can be simulated by subjecting collagenous structures to cyclic loading and unloading programmes. Rigby (1964) carried out experiments of this nature on tendons and deduced from the diffraction pattern that subjection to stretching cycles results in an increased degree of orientation.

Elastin

Elastic fibres are not as highly oriented as collagen fibres, and X-ray diffraction patterns for elastin are restricted to relatively diffuse concentric halos, the diameters of which are consonant with units repeating every 0.22 and 0.44–0.45 nm, and others which lie about 0.9 nm apart (Cox and Little, 1961). In his introduction to a symposium on connective tissue held in 1957 (Tunbridge, 1958), Astbury suggested that the X-ray diffraction pattern of elastin, which is in many ways similar to that of thermally denatured collagen, may indicate that elastin is a member of the collagen group of proteins which has a thermal denaturation temperature below that of the normal mammalian body temperature. It would appear more likely, however, that the distortion of the molecules in the elastic fibres into the amorphous non-crystalline state in which it exists, is brought about by the interaction of terminal aldehyde and amino groups which originate from lysine residues (cf. p. 87). The formation of tri- and quadridentate desmosine molecules draws together adjacent polypeptide chains and disturbs the potential crystallinity of the elastic structure. This formation of cross-linkages can be shown to be age determined in so far as the number of free ε-amino groups on the lysine residues is far greater in foetal than in adult tissues. No marked changes occur however, during advanced ageing, and the phenomenon may be regarded as being one which is more closely associated with maturation than with ageing *per se*.

Electron microscopic evidence for age changes

Collagen

The major fibrous components of connective tissue can be identified in the electron microscope either in teased specimens (Wyckoff and Corey, 1936; Wolpers, 1944), in thin section (Rhodin and Dalham, 1955), in the scanning electron microscope (Hunter and Finlay, 1973) or after freeze-etching (Reed, 1973). The scanning electron microscope is most useful for the study of the fine details of superficial tissue structure and may be regarded as providing a high resolution extension in three dimensions of the structural evidence which can be obtained from light microscopic studies. The other three variations of electron microscopy permit the microstructure of the fibrils to be examined with resolving powers of between 0.1 and 0.5 nm. At this level, collagen can be seen to consist of micro-fibrils between 10 and 250 nm in diameter (Schwarz, 1957). In general, the fibrils increase in diameter with increasing age. For instance, the median diameter of foetal achilles tendon collagen is 35 nm. By 4 years of age this has increased to 45 nm and by 42 years the distribution of fibre diameter is bimodal, with a lower peak still at 40–50 nm, but with some

40% of the fibres having diameters around 100 nm. Coupled with this increase in fibre diameter is a marked dispersion of the size distribution, even in tissues in which a bimodal distribution does not develop with age. In the rat tail tendon for instance (Schwarz, 1957), (Fig. 31) the range of diameters increases from 20–100 nm at 4 weeks to 30–200 nm by 1 year. Linke (1955) has reported, however, that the fibrils of the skin grow thinner in extreme old age. Keech (1961), studying the appearance in the electron microscope of collagen fibrils regenerated from solution observed that the presence of chondroitin sulphate in the precipitating medium greatly increased the rate at which collagen fibrils were formed, and lowered the diameter of the fibrils by a factor of 3. The newly regenerated fibrils with which she was dealing were between 200 and 240 nm in diameter in control preparations, and on the addition of CSA the diameters fell to between 70 and 100 nm. Wood (1960, 1964) has shown that the rate of

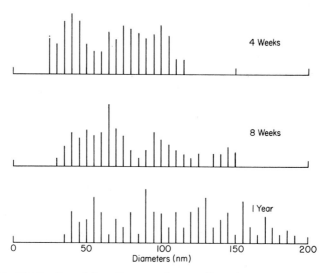

FIG. 31. The distribution of fibre diameters in rat tail tendon at 4 weeks, 8 weeks and 1 year of age.

reconstitution of collagen fibrils and hence their diameter, is related not only to the presence or absence of polyanions, such as chrondroitin sulphate, but also to their chemical structure. Thus chondroitin 4 and 6 sulphates initiate rapid fibril formation and the presence of such compounds in high concentration in a tissue could result in fine fibril formation, whereas hyaluronic acid, dermatan sulphate and keratan sulphate do not affect the precipitation rate and may be expected to permit the lateral alignment of tropocollagen molecules to give broader fibrils. Both qualitative and quantitative differences in the glycosaminoglycan content of various tissues may, therefore, determine the nature of the collagen network which is laid down, but equally important from the age point of view is the fact that the nature of the glycosaminoglycan in any one tissue may change with age (cf. p. 138). If the tissue concerned is one in which a certain degree of remodelling, with removal and resynthesis of collagen fibres, can occur throughout life, it is possible that any fibres laid down in maturity and old age may be appreciably different in diameter to those laid down in youth. As has been shown earlier in the section on mechanical properties, the rigidity and elasticity of a tissue depends as much on the number of fibres which constitute its bulk as on the total mass of collagen which is present. Hence alterations in fibre diameter may have a marked effect on the physical properties and function of the tissue.

Collagen fibrils in normal adult tissues can be characterised in the electron microscope by the presence of regularly spaced cross striations. When the tissue, either teased apart or sectioned, is coated with metal to enhance its structural characteristics, the fibrils can be seen to consist of a longitudinal series of regions of greater or less density and diameter, the distance between crests measuring from 64 to 70 nm (Schmitt *et al.*, 1942). If, on the other hand, the tissue preparations are stained with electron dense metal-containing stains which attach themselves specifically to the polar regions of the molecules, the light and dark or thick and thin areas of the fibrils can be split into up to 14 subsidiary bands (Fig. 32). The distribution of these bands is not symmetrical but polarised, and each band is repeated every 65–70 nm, thus

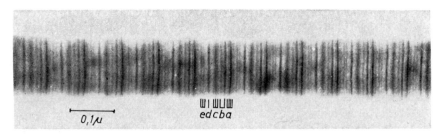

edcba

0,1μ

FIG. 32. Electron micrograph of collagen microfibril stained with phosphotunystic acid showing fine detail in the striations.

indicating that it is the repetition of these individual charged centres which determines the overall characteristic periodicity of the collagen fibril. Over the past 20 years studies on this naturally occurring form of collagen and on other artificially produced forms; fibrous long spacing (FLS) (Highberger *et al.*, 1950) and segment long spacing (SLS) (Schmitt *et al.*, 1953) has enabled the tertiary structure of the fibres to be elucidated, and it has been demonstrated that naturally occurring collagen consists of an assembly of rigid tropocollagen molecules. Each of these, measuring approximately 280 by 1.4 nm and having a molecular weight of 360 000 daltons, is arranged relative to adjacent molecules so that they overlap one another by 210 nm, i.e. by three quarters of their length. It has recently been suggested (Smith, 1968; Hodge and Petrushka, 1963) that each tropocollagen molecule may be divided into four equal sections and a fifth smaller section. The four equal lengths (D) are each equivalent to a characteristic 64 nm period and the shorter, terminal portion is 0.4 D (i.e. 25.6 nm). Allowing for the staggered overlap this means that a gap of 0.6 D (38.4 nm) lies between each longitudinal pair of tropocollagen molecules. The present consensus of opinion is therefore, contrary to the earlier concept that each collagen fibril consists of a lateral array of microfibrils formed by the longitudinal aggregation of tropocollagen molecules. It is in fact in favour of the suggestion that the integrity of the fibril as a whole is dependent on lateral cross-linkage between individual tropocollagen molecules, which are longitudinally independent of one another. Early electron microscope studies in which the fibrils themselves were mounted, shadowed or stained and examined, could only permit the measurement of the dimensions of dried fibrils, since the tissue was dehydrated after its introduction into the vacuum chamber of the microscope. Under these conditions the repeating period was 64 nm. More recent studies, in which replication techniques have been employed, have permitted measurements to be made on fibrils which still retain their characteristic amount of moisture. Under these conditions the repeating period is extended to 68 nm, i.e. by an amount which is appreciably less than the gap between longitudinally adjacent tropocollagen molecules. The cross-linkages which bind the tropocollagen molecules to their laterally placed neighbours (either hydrogen or co-valent bonds) are sufficiently strong to withstand any further swelling which might occur as the result of the introduction of larger amounts of water. As the number and complexity of the cross-linkage between adjacent molecules increases with increasing age, it would be expected that the permissible longitudinal as well as the lateral displacements would decrease, and this would prevent the fibres from swelling when exposed to moisture either in the form of water vapour or liquid. It is, therefore, significant that the moisure content of collagen from old tissues is lower than that of collagen from young tissues (Meyer, 1931).

In foetal tissue or in fibrils immediately after synthesis in tissue culture, the characteristic periodicity is not the 65–70 nm typical of mature fibres, but 21–22 nm. This appears to represent one of the first stages in the formation of the tertiary structure of the collagen macromolecule. Arising from studies of the skin of dermatosparaxic cattle (Lapierre et al., 1971) it has been shown (Martin, 1972) that the individual α-chains, as synthesised on the polysomes of the fibroblasts, contain 20% extra terminal peptide regions which are not characteristic of the collagen molecule as it exists extracellularly. These peptides on each of the so-called pro-α-chains assist in their alignment to form procollagen molecules in which the individual chains are wound round one another in a helical structure. Following glycosylation the extraneous terminal polypeptide is removed by an enzyme, procollagen protease, and secreted by the cell. Veis (1972) has suggested that this removal of the procollagen peptide, may occur in a series of stages, and it may be that the retention of part of the procollagen peptide in the extracellular environment prevents the quarter stagger alignment of tropocollagen molecules which is typical of mature collagen, and constrains a closer degree of packing which results in the 21–22 nm periodicity seen in collagen immediately after synthesis. Although the development of the truly mature 65–70 nm form from this primitive structure is time dependent, the conversion can hardly be classified as an ageing phenomenon since it occurs primarily in the very earliest period of life. It does, however, provide a base line from which it is possible to assess the relative stability of the mature collagen fibre, since the latter retains its characteristic 65–70 nm periodicity unchanged until the death of the organism.

Degradation of collagen with age

Although the 65–70 nm periodicity is still apparent in tissues of great age, other changes do occur, which result in the destruction of the whole structure of the fibril. This degradation of collagenous structures can be observed in a number of ageing tissues, and is also apparent in a variety of pathological conditions, but the most well documented changes are those which accompany the ageing and exposure to ultra-violet irradiation of skin.

Tunbridge *et al.* (1950) first studied samples of tissue from the exposed surfaces of the forearms of elderly subjects in the electron microscope, and observed that material from regions of skin which, on the basis of histological examination, would appear to have suffered marked elastosis, did not in fact contain high concentrations of elastic fibres, but were rich in broken and degenerate collagen fibres (Fig. 19). In any normal electron microscope field, even of teased tissue, it is unusual to see cut or broken fibril ends. All the fibrils extend across the complete field. In the case of preparations from exposed elderly dermis, the lengths of fibre are visibly shorter, with many acute breaks and bends and they are all covered with a mass of amorphous debris which partially obscures their characteristic cross striations. Hall (1968a) has suggested that the name pseudoelastin, which had originally been ascribed to altered collagen on the basis of its tinctorial properties (Gillman *et al.*, 1955a, b) should be given to the degenerate collagen identified in this way in the dermis. Further work on the chemical identity of this protein has proved its relationship to collagen, although its tinctorial properties are closely akin to those of elastin (Hall, 1964), (p. 103).

Degradation of a protein constituent of connective tissue must imply the existence of proteolytic enzymes capable of bringing about the disruption of the polypeptide chains. It has recently been shown (review by Evanson, 1976) that such enzyme systems, capable of digesting collagen, are present in a number of connective tissues, but studies on the effect of microbiological collagenases on collagens from tissues of various ages had previously demonstrated that material with the appearance of pseudoelastin could be produced in collagenous tissues.

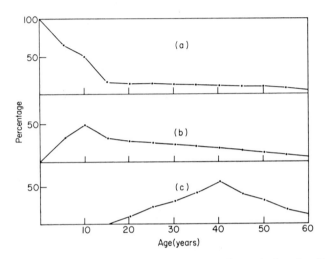

FIG. 33. The distribution of various degradation products during the digestion of human skin collagens of varying age. (a) Granular degeneration – the overall disruption of the fibrils into particulate material. (b) Pseudoelastin production (c) Standard form of degradation – the breakdown of individual microfibrils into tactoids. (cf. Fig. 43.)

Keech (1954a, b, 1955) showed that the effect of *Clostridium histolyticum* collagenase on collagen varied markedly with increasing age (Fig. 33). She divided the products of extensive collagenase action into three major groups, on the basis of their appearance in the electron microscope. The progressive degradation of the collagen fibres under the action of collagenase produced either shorter fibrils with tapered ends, or granular deposits, which appeared to develop uniformly throughout the tissue. Tapered ends were typical of the degradation of fibres derived from all subjects above 30 years of age, while granular degeneration occurred in fibres from subjects up to 20 years of age. Between 10 and 35 years of age, however, a third type of degradation product was evident, consisting of broad irregular masses of electron dense tissue. Not only was this material resistant to further attack by collagenase, it was also resistant to gelatinisation when placed in boiling water, whereas the tapered fibrils and the granular residue from old and young tissues respectively were both easily transformed into highly swollen gelatinous masses on heating. Keech later reported that these masses of amorphous material could be produced in the absence of any digestive enzyme by treatment for relatively short periods, (1–6 h at 37° C) with 1% sodium periodate, pH 5, or for slightly longer (24 h) with pH 8.8 borate buffer (Keech *et al.*, 1956).

Some confusion arose in the literature since Keech, observing the greater degree of similarity between elastin and the degraded form of collagen which resulted from partial digestion or treatment with buffer, referred to "the conversion of collagen to 'elastin' ". In her papers, and in those which dealt with the biochemical changes which accompanied partial degradation of collagen (Burton *et al.*, 1955; Hall *et al.*, 1955; Hall and Tunbridge, 1957; Hall, 1956) no claim was made that this material was identical with naturally occurring elastin, although the authors were at pains to point out that it demonstrated many of the properties of elastin. Similar material was reported by Banga and Balo (1956) following thermal or chemical denaturation of tendon collagen and called by them metacollagen, whereas Tustanovsky *et al.* (1954) reported similar properties for the material which they isolated from collagenous tissues after the removal of the soluble form of the collagen, and to which they gave the name collastromin.

In other tissues and as the result of a variety of pathological conditions (Hall, 1973b) pseudoelastins of different appearance have been identified. This demonstrates that rather than classify all forms of pseudoelastin as identical it would be more appropriate to refer to a *group* of pseudoelastins representing a variety of stages in the degradation of collagen.

Elastin

Elastin from mature tissues shows no evidence of microstructure (Fig. 34), unless prolonged staining is resorted to (Cliff, 1971) but in elastin from foetal tissue, numerous microfibrillar elements can be observed (Fig. 35) (Ross and Bornstein, 1969). It has recently been demonstrated (Ross, 1973) that the presence of such material in appreciable concentration is associated with the appearance of relatively large amounts of structural glycoproteins (cf. p. 136), and it has been deduced that this indicates that these microfibrillar elements, around which the elastin is deposited during maturation, are glycoprotein in nature. It has also been shown that the regions immediately under the plaques in an arteriosclerotic aortic wall are rich in glycoprotein. This may indicate *de novo* elastin synthesis in these areas, but there is no evidence as yet that the glycoprotein which is laid down in atherosclerosis is in a fibrillar form. It may be that glycoprotein which occurs in aged and atherosclerotic aorta is similar in composition to the amorphous pseudoelastin which has also been observed under these conditions.

Kadar *et al.* (1973) have reported that the microfibrils of elastic tissue

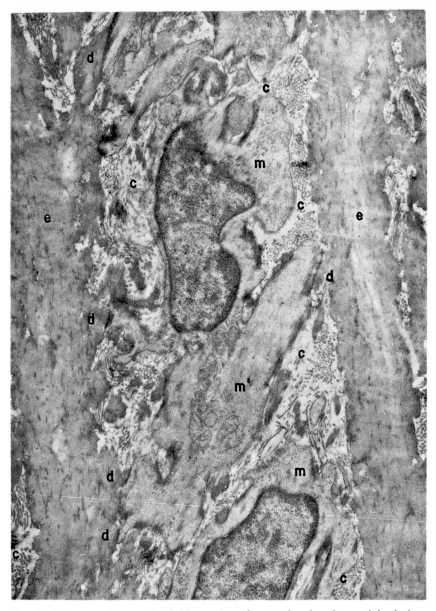

FIG. 34. Electron micrograph of thin section of aorta showing the spatial relationship between elastin (e), collagen (c) and smooth muscle (m). The regions labelled (d) are points of attachment of the elastin and muscle. ($\times$ 15 000)

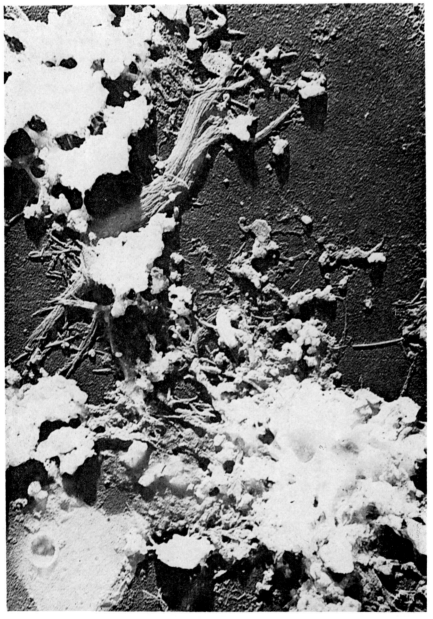

FIG. 35. Electron micrograph of teased sample of aortic elastin, showing the amorphous protein elastin, and the glycoprotein fibrils. (×0000)

consist of a beaded structure 12 nm in diameter, on which globular particles 18 nm in diameter are superimposed. In this respect, these structures bear a close resemblance to those observed by Hall et al. (1955) as the penultimate product of elastolysis. The elastase preparations employed during these early studies were by no means pure, and it is quite probable that they contained non-specific proteolytic enzymes, such as trypsin. It is not surprising, therefore, that at that time it was reported that these particulate microfibrils were also dissolved, although similar structures present in the microfibrillar portion of the elastin fibre have recently been shown to be resistant to attack by the purer preparations of elastase now available.

4

Chemical and Biochemical Changes in Ageing Connective Tissues

Collagen

The collagen content of ageing tissues

The amounts of collagen present in any given tissue is dependent on the simultaneous activity of anabolic (Little and Valderrama, 1964) and catabolic (Burrows, 1965) systems. These two effects are dealt with separately elsewhere in this volume (pp. 165 and 169) but overall values are of interest *per se* since the actual amount of collagen present in a tissue at any one time is of importance in determining the physical properties of the tissue as a whole.

Skin. Harris and Sjoerdsma (1966) reported little change in the collagen content of human dermis between the ages of 19 and 40 years, the range of values being from 95 to 129 mg/g dry tissue. Fleischmajer *et al.* (1973) studying a larger number of subjects over a wider age range (birth to 96 years of age) also provided no evidence for age changes, although their results were slightly lower than those of Harris and Sjoerdsma (ranging from 92 to 106 mg/g dry weight of tissue). This method for recording collagen content takes no account of the possibility of changes in the total mass of the dermis. Skin thickness can be measured with spring loaded Harpenden calipers or by a radiological method (Sheppard and Meema, 1967). The results obtained by these two methods are not in complete agreement, Sheppard and Meema for instance, observing no significant alteration in skin thickness with age whereas McConkey *et al.* (1963), Rychewaert (1967) and Meema *et al.* at an earlier date, 1964, using the caliper method observed decreases in skin thickness in human dermis above the age of 45 in females and 55 in males. Shuster and Bottoms (1963) and Reed and Hall (1974) used a method for recording the relative amounts of collagen in the dermis of subjects of varying age which employed measurements of collagen content/mm² of skin surface. Samples of skin of a fixed area were removed from the leg of living subjects, care being taken to include the whole thickness of the dermis. In this way the whole of the collagen beneath one square millimetre of skin surface could be calculated,

79

instead of the concentration of collagen as calculated by Harris and Sjoerd-sma's method.

Shuster and Bottoms (1967) reported a reduction in total skin collagen with age, but this was not confirmed by Reed and Hall (1974). Hall *et al.* (1974), however, did observe a fall with age and confirmed Shuster and Bottoms' finding that the amount of collagen present in skin was at all ages higher in males than females. Hall *et al.* (1974) recorded a reduction of 136 μg/mm^2/year in the collagen content of the skin of female subjects, but the scatter was so great that the *P* value for a regression line of this slope was only 0.02; barely significant.

The cardiovascular system. The collagen content of the cardiovascular system has been studied by numerous workers, since although in certain vessels elastin represents the major portion of the tissue, in all the collagen component is of considerable importance in determining the response of the tissue to the pressures invoked by blood flow.

Harkness *et al.* (1957) have examined the collagen content of the arteries of dogs, and have shown that in the intrathoracic aorta the major component is elastin, and the collagen content never rises above 35%. In other vessels, however, the collagen content may be as high as 70%. Berry and Looker (1973) and Berry *et al.* (1972) have recorded the amounts of collagen in the aortas of rats ranging in age from the tenth week of foetal growth to one year of age. In the period of antenatal growth the collagen content of the aorta rises from 28 to between 37 and 40% of the dry fat-free weight, but after birth there appears to be no further significant increase. As a proportion of the total scleroprotein content (collagen and elastin combined) the collagen continues to rise with age since the elastin levels falls very slightly. Banga (1969) gave values for the absolute collagen content and the proportion which this substance formed of the total scleroprotein, in the aortas of human subjects, ranging in age from 16 to 90. Being an unselected population of human subjects many of the older ones showed frank signs of arteriosclerosis, and hence the possibility of correlating any alterations in collagen with age itself was not high. The values she obtained varied considerably depending on the method used for analysis, and ranged from 28 to 81% over the age range 17 to 76 if the elastin was removed by elastolysis, and from 17 to 32% if the collagen was assessed by measurement of the hydroxyproline contents of hydrolysates of whole tissue. In view of the very varied causes of death recorded for these subjects, it is not surprising that there appears to be no overall age related change in collagen content. Even comparing subjects with a minimal degree of arteriosclerosis as assessed by WHO standards, there is no significant trend with age.

Dagliotti (1931) could find little change in the collagen content of the ventricular connective tissue, an observation which was confirmed by Lev and McMillan (1961) and McMillan and Lev (1962). Ehrenberg *et al.* (1954), however, reported that the collagen content of the ventrical increased with age, a change which according to Lev and McMillan was restricted to the atrium. All these observations were made by a quantification of histological studies, but chemical determinations were equally if not more inconclusive. Blumgart *et al.* (1940) and Montfort and Perez-Tamayo (1962) found no variation with age. Oken and Boucek (1957) and Wegelius and von Knorring (1964) observed a decrease, whilst Clausen (1962) reported a steady increase in collagen levels with increasing age.

The biochemical findings on average gave values for the collagen content which were between 3 and 9 % of those obtained by the histochemical methods. Lenkiewicz *et al.* (1972) employed a flying spot scanner to automate a histological procedure, and although the errors which are inherent in all histological methods still remain, the removal of the human factor renders their results more acceptable. The percentage of the volume of the interventricular septum which stains as collagen rises from around 22 % in the early teens to either 27 or 31 % at the age of 90 depending on the orientation of the fibres. Areas in which the muscle fibres were predominantly longitudinal to the section gave the lower values in old age.

The skeleton. The loss of collagen from bony tissue is associated with a loss of calcium phosphate as well as contributing to the condition known as osteoporosis. This is dealt with in more detail elsewhere (p. 52) and is shown to consist of a truly age-determined phenomena on which is superimposed under certain pathological conditions an excessive loss of bone mass, and hence collagenous bone matrix, over and above that which is typical of the age group concerned.

The fundamental structure of the collagen molecule

In young connective tissues, collagen consists of an array of protein chains arranged in a series of triple helices – the tropocollagen molecules – held together by hydrogen bonds. X-ray diffraction studies and electron-microscopic examination demonstrate how these molecules are aligned relative to one another (p. 67), but it is the fundamental amino and imino acid composition of the molecules themselves which determines how this is accomplished.

The central portion of each molecular chain consists of 1012 amino and imino acid residues. These are not arranged throughout in a sequence consisting exclusively of a repeating series of triads, as was originally thought to be the case (Shroeder *et al.*, 1953), but the proportion of proline and hydroxyproline taken together is approximately half that of the total of the other amino acids and in many sequences an imino acid does occupy every third site. The other sites in the chain may be occupied either by hydroxyproline residues (where the third residue is proline) or by neutral or polar amino acids. Regions exist which are rich in hydroxyproline, and others which are rich in polar amino acids, and the two areas are mutually exclusive. Chapman (1974) has shown that the displacement of adjacent chains relative to one another by 233 residues, i.e. by a value for this displacement period, D, equalling $0.22 \times$ the length of the tropocollagen molecule (as opposed to the figure of $0.25\ L$ deduced from electron microscope studies (cf. p. 72) results in an alignment of those regions which are rich in polar amino acids into twelve bands which repeat every $0.22\ L$ along the length of the molecule. Ninety per cent of the individual polar residues can be included in these polar amino acid-rich sections of the molecule which correspond in position to those regions of the fibril, which can be shown in the electron microscope to stain with uranyl acetate and phosphotungstic acid and which have been named the SLS interperiod bands a_1 to e_2 (Fig. 32) (Bruns and Gross, 1973).

At the N- and C-terminal ends of the polypeptide chains are short lengths of peptide, the so-called *telopeptide* regions which neither contain hydroxyproline, nor are twisted into the helical configuration which characterises the rest of the molecule. The N-terminal telopeptide is 15 residues in length, whereas the C-terminal end consists of 25 residues (Fig. 36). There are four polar residues in each telopeptide and of these the lysine residues can form the basis of inter-chain linkages.

N-terminal telopeptide of 1-chain of collagen
Glu–Met–Ser–Tyr–Gly–Tyr–Asp–Glu–Lys–Ser–Ala–Gly–Val–Ser–Pro–

C-terminal telopeptide of 1-chain of collagen
Tyr–Tyr–Arg–Gly–Gly–Asp–His–Lys–Glx–Gln–Gln–
–Pro–Pro–Gln–Pro–Leu–Phe–Ser–Leu–Asp–Try–Gly–Gly–Ser

FIG. 36. The amino acid sequence of the N- and C-terminal telopeptides of the collagen molecule.

The details presented above are those for only one species of polypeptide chain, the so-called α1-chain. Studies on collagens from various sites have indicated the presence of a different α2-chain which has a quite dissimilar amino acid analysis. Moreover, in certain non-vertebrate collagens tropocollagen may consist of three slightly dissimilar α1-chains. Since the tropocollagen molecule is formed by the helical arrangement of the three α-chains, there are four possible combinations of α-chain, which can make up the trihelical molecule $((\alpha 1)_3; (\alpha 1)_2 \alpha 2; \alpha 1(\alpha 2)_2$ and $(\alpha 2)_3)$ and these have been identified in various tissues (Table 1).

Immediately after synthesis (see below) the tropocollagen triple helix is stabilised by hydrogen bonds formed between the peptide groupings of one polypeptide chain and a hydroxyl group in an adjacent chain. The presently accepted structure for the collagen molecule presupposes that the maximum number of hydrogen bonds are formed and that the alignment of each bond will be as nearly co-planar with the groupings it links together as is possible. These criteria have permitted the elimination of a number of theoretically possible structures (Ramachandran, 1963) and have pointed clearly to the Rich and Crick model No. II (Rich and Crick, 1955, 1958, 1961) as being the most probable. Such hydrogen bonds, although strong enough to retain the collagen molecules in place in the tissue under normal physiological conditions, are easily broken, either by the swelling forces which arise when the collagen becomes heavily hydrated following the ionisation of the polar groupings in the molecule in acidic or alkaline media, or if the fibre should be immersed in solutions of hydrogen bond breaking reagents such as urea, thiocyanate or guanidine. Denaturation, resulting in the separation of the individual α-chains, can also be accomplished by the elevation of the temperature of the neutral aqueous medium in which the collagen is suspended, to 40 °C. Following denaturation, foetal and infant collagenous structures can be completely fractionated into the component α-chains by chromatography on cationic ionexchange cellulose columns (Miller, 1976) or by gel-electrophoresis (Clark, 1976).

TABLE 1. Distribution of collagen α-chains in various tissues.

α-chain composition	
$[\alpha 1(I)]_2 \alpha 2$	Dermis, tendon, bone
$[\alpha 1(II)]_3$	Cartilage
$[\alpha 1(III)]_3$	Dermis, aorta
$[\alpha 1(IV)]_3$	Basement, membrane lens

At later stages of development other denaturation products of the extracttable collagen are apparent in the eluates from carboxy-methyl-cellulose columns or in gel-electrophoresis slabs (Heikkinen and Kulonen, 1964) (Fig. 37). The amounts of collagen extractable with neutral salt or acid buffers also change with age, falling to quite low levels by the time maturity is attained. Heikkinen and Kulonen (1964) have for instance examined the species of collagen molecules which are extracted by solutions of neutral salt from the skins of rats ranging in age from 6 weeks to 24 months, using starch-gel electrophoresis (Fig. 38) and have shown that the proportion of the

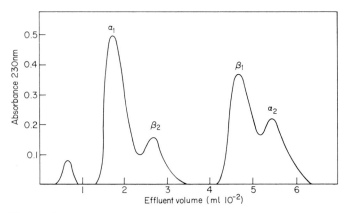

FIG. 37. Elution diagram of the components of denatured soluble collagen separated on a carboxymethyl cellulose column.

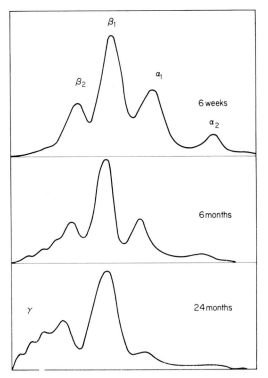

FIG. 38. The distribution of α-chains and other species of collagen in rat skins of various ages. Calculated from the observations of Heikkinen and Kulonen (1964).

collagen which is extractable in the form of free α-chains, decreases with age; whereas the amounts of the larger molecules, α-chain dimers (β-collagen) and trimers (γ-collagen) increase. In fact, however, an examination of the areas of the densitometry peaks recorded by these workers (Hall, 1973a) shows that it is the trimeric and larger polymers of tropocollagen which increase with age at the expense of the free α-chains whilst the dimeric forms remain roughly constant (Table 2).

TABLE 2. Age changes in the percentage monomeric and polymeric composition of soluble collagen in skin tissue from rats, calculated from the densitometric assessment of starch-gel electropherograms. (Heikkinen and Kulonen, 1964.)

Type of collagen	Age (months)				
	1.5	*3*	*6*	*12*	*24*
α	40	43	37	22	19
β	54	54	54	54	54
γ*	2	3	9	24	27

* Refers to trimeric and larger molecular species of collagen.

Bornstein *et al.* (1964) have shown that in tissues containing two $\alpha 1$ and one $\alpha 2$-chains forms of the β and γ polymers of collagen exist, which can only be explained on the assumption that *inter* as well as *intra*molecular co-valent bonds are formed as the tissue matures. Thus for instance, in tissues in which the distribution of α-chains is one $\alpha 2$ to two $\alpha 1$, *intra*molecular linkages could only result in the formation of β_{11} and and β_{12} dimers and γ_{112} trimers. Bornstein and Piez (1964) and Veis and Anesy (1965), however, observed the presence of β_{22}, γ_{122} and γ_{222} species which could only have been derived as the result of cross-linkages between adjacent tropocollagen molecules, and moreover by linkages which formed preferentially between $\alpha 2$-chains (see also p. 89).

Not only do the tropocollagen molecules themselves become more stable as cross-linkages develop, but the microfibrils as well are less easily dissolved or metabolised as the formation of linkages between adjacent collagen molecules proceeds.

The nature of the cross-linkages of the collagen molecule

Introduction. The mass of information which is now available regarding the nature, number and distribution of cross-links in the collagen molecule and their change with age may be said to have originated with the hypotheses of Verzar (1963) and Bjorksten (1958) regarding the ageing of connective tissues. Verzar (p. 21) reported increasing degrees of resistance to thermal contraction with increasing age, in the case of rat-tail tendon, and Bjorksten based his deductions on a study of the changing solubility and resistance to enzymic attack which occurs with increasing age.

A logical deduction from this evidence of increasing structural and bio-chemical stability is that the individual polypeptide chains in the collagen molecule, and possibly the molecules themselves are more closely bound to one another as age progresses, but at that time in the late 1950s and early 1960s nothing was known of the chemical nature of these proposed cross-linkages. Since then, their existence has been confirmed and details of their structure determined by partial hydrolysis, purification and analysis. Over the past 5–10 years details of the primary, secondary and tertiary structures of collagen and their change with age, have become increasingly clear and knowledge regarding the maturation processes of the molecules has developed.

The biosynthesis of collagen. Certain of the modifications which take place in the molecule as it is originally synthesised cannot be regarded as being age-mediated since they occur early in the biosynthesis of all collagen fibrils, at whatever stage they are produced in the life of the organism. The completion of these modifications, however, is essential for such subsequent changes as are age-mediated, and hence an understanding of their nature is imperative before the age changes *per se* can be appreciated.

The polypeptide chains of collagen are synthesised as the result of enzymic processes acting at ribosomal-messenger RNA complexes within the cyto-plasm of connective tissue fibroblasts (Gould, 1968a, b), but this RNA is not programmed for the incorporation of the two residues typical of collagen – hydroxyproline and hydroxylysine (Stetten and Schoenheimer, 1944; Stetten, 1949). The sites ultimately to be filled by these residues are initially filled by proline and lysine residues respectively. Hydroxylation takes place sub-sequently under the control of specific enzymes, namely protocollagen and lysine hydroxylases (Adams, 1970). The individual polypeptides, with molecu-lar weights of about 120 000 daltons are large when compared with other nascent proteins and the m-RNA chain responsible for the selection and introduction of the 1000 or more amino and imino acids must be large by normal standards. It was believed at one stage in the development of informa-tion regarding collagen structure and biosynthesis (Gallop *et al.*, 1959) that the individual α-chains consisted of sub-subunits joined together by non-peptide linkages. This would have permitted smaller polypeptide elements to be synthesised on separate m-RNA molecules; these small molecules then being united through ester links by other systems not under ribosomal control. This concept has now been shown to be incorrect, each α-chain consisting of a single continuous polypeptide unit requiring an m-RNA molecule of dimensions which are sufficiently large for its synthesis. Recently Lazarides and Lukens (1971) have shown that the size of the m-RNA molecule in chick embryo fibroblasts does in fact correspond in size to that required to code for a single chain, fully 1000 or more residues in length.

Until recently it was not known how the alignment of the α-chains was accomplished to produce the triple helical structure of the tropocollagen molecule. However, Dehm et al. (1972) have shown that immediately after synthesis the polypeptide chain is some 13 nm longer than the mature α-chain, and it has been suggested that these extra N-terminal peptides which contain cysteine residues can react with one another through the oxidation of pairs of thiol groups in adjacent chains to form cystine cross-linkages. These locate the pro-α-chains relative to one another, permitting helix formation with the production of pro-collagen. The excess terminal peptide region is then removed either at the cell membrane or immediately extracellularly by the action of a specialised peptidase(s) (Lapierre et al., 1971; Bornstein et al., 1972). Bornstein (1972) has suggested that once helix formation has occurred, part at least of the N-terminal registration peptide is removed within the cell, further hydrolysis to tropocollagen occurring after or during extrusion through the membrane.

Lysine based cross-links. As the tropocollagen molecule matures, the "non-covalent hydrophic electrostatic and hydrogen bonds" (Bailey and Robins, 1973) which initially hold the molecules together are augmented by the introduction of various types of co-valent linkage.

A variety of possible reactive groups has been proposed for the initiation of the cross-linkages both between the individual α-chains and between tropocollagen molecules, but the existence of aldehyde groups has proved to be of prime importance, and it has been shown that these are derived by the oxidative deamination of lysine residues.

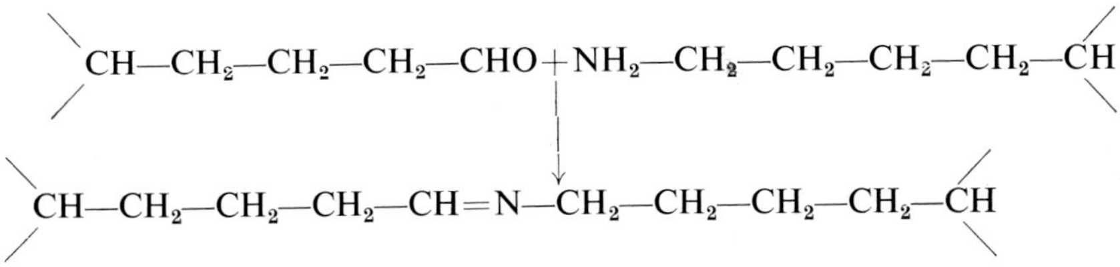

$$\begin{array}{c}\diagdown\\ CH-CH_2-CH_2-CH_2-CHO + NH_2-CH_2-CH_2-CH_2-CH_2-CH \diagup \\ \diagup \qquad\qquad\qquad\qquad\qquad\qquad\qquad\qquad\qquad \diagdown \\ \big| \\ \downarrow \\ \diagdown \\ CH-CH_2-CH_2-CH_2-CH=N-CH_2-CH_2-CH_2-CH_2-CH \diagup \\ \diagup \qquad\qquad\qquad\qquad\qquad\qquad\qquad\qquad\qquad \diagdown \end{array}$$

Fig. 39. The formation of a Schiff's base by the condensation of one molecule of allysine and one molecule of lysine.

Levene and Gross (1950), studying lathyrism induced by the administration of β-amino proprionitrile to chick embryos, demonstrated that the aldehyde content of lathyritic collagen was markedly reduced. The possible role of aldehydes in cross-linkage formation in connective tissue proteins was subsequently deduced from studies of elastin cross-links (Thomas et al., 1963) (see p. 121). Fessler and Bailey (1965) suggested that the aldehydes might react with amino groups to form Schiff's bases between adjacent chains. They reduced the Schiff's bases or aldimines with (Fig. 39) boro-hydride, to stabilise them so that they would resist destruction during attempts to separate cross-linked peptide elements following dilute acid hydrolysis. Reduction however, also stabilised the intact fibril against attack by dilute acids and α-amino thiols (Bailey, 1967; Tanzer, 1968), thus confirming the existence of reducible bonds not only between the individual α-chains, but also between adjacent tropocollagen molecules.

The studies which have been made on lathyrism have enabled the first stage of the cross-linking reaction to be elucidated. Pinnell and Martin (1968) detected an enzyme system, lysine oxidase, in embryonic chick bone, which is capable of removing the ϵ-amino group and oxidising the ϵ-carbon atom of protein-bound lysine residues. The resulting residue of δ-amino adipic acid semi aldehyde-allysine can be shown to increase at the expense of protein bound lysine. Free lysine cannot be deaminated in this fashion, thus indicating that the enzyme is distinct from other forms of monoamino oxidase, such as that present in plasma. The system is inhibited by levels of β-aminopropionitrile (βAPN) which have little effect on other amino oxidases, but which Levene and Gross (1959) have shown to be capable of inhibiting cross-link formation in collagen *in vivo*. Several authors have suggested that there is a close similarity between the connective tissue disorders associated with experimental lathyrism and copper deficiency. Shields *et al.*, 1962; Miller *et al.*, 1965; Piez, 1968 and Siegel *et al.*, 1970, have demonstrated that this is in fact the case. βAPN could prevent cross-link formation and thus initiate tissue disorders, by blocking that stage of the reaction at which the allysine residue from one tropocollagen molecule condenses with either an aldehyde or an amino group in another chain. This would explain for instance how this semicarbazide and various hydrazines act as lathyritic agents, since they are capable of reacting with aldehyde groups. The reduction in the amounts of aldehyde group present in lathyritic and copper deficient collagen and elastin, however, indicates that the lesion most probably originates at the first step in cross-link formation, i.e. the actual oxidative production of the allysine residue. Pinnell and Martin (1968) observed that lysyl oxidase is inactivated following incubation with βAPN *in vitro* probably by the formation of a copper complex which is similar in its non-effectiveness as a metal co-factor for the enzyme to that produced by chelating agents such as $\alpha\alpha'$-dipyridyl. It is possible to demonstrate (Hall, unpublished observations) that all the potentially lathyrogenic reagents reported by Levene and Gross (1950) form complexes with copper which can be identified by a shift of the copper absorption peak to a lower wavelength, between 230 and 320 nm. Whether these complexes are sufficiently strong to withdraw the copper entirely from the enzyme system has not as yet been proved. Levene (1961) is however, of the opinion that chelation of copper cannot provide a full explanation of the lathyritic activity of reagents as varied as nitriles, ureides, hydrazides and hydrazines.

The next stage in the formation of cross-links from lysine-derived aldehydes may be under the control of other enzyme systems, but it may also be a spontaneous reaction. Solutions of collagen precipitate on standing (Gross, 1963) and this may be due to the spontaneous formation of covalent linkages by the interaction of protein bound aldehydes either with other aldehydes or with amines. Confirmation of this can be obtained from a consideration of the fact that the gel/sol interconversion of aldehyde-deficient collagen from lathyritic tissues remains reversible when the pH or temperature is returned to the levels at which freshly prepared gels from normal tissue repass into solution (Nimni, 1966).

Sites of cross-linkage. In general the introduction of an aldehyde group into a collagen molecule occurs most readily at the lysine residues located nine residues from the N-terminus of the α1-chain (Traub and Piez, 1971) and in position 6 in the α2-chain. Rauterberg and Kuhn (1971) and Rauterberg *et al.* (1972) have however also identified allysine in the 1044th residue, i.e. the ninth residue from the end of the C-terminal telopeptide. The other ends of the cross-links have been located by CNBr fractionation in various positions throughout the length of the trihelical portion of the molecule. Treatment with this reagent cleaves the molecule at each methionine residue, breaking it into eight peptides of varying length (Bornstein and Piez, 1966). Allowing for the $0.22D$ stagger (cf. p. 82) and the short overlap zone (Smith, 1968; Miller and Wray, 1972) it can be assumed that the N-terminal telopeptide of one α-chain (either α1 or α2) will be cross-linked either with the fifth or sixth CNBr fraction of an α1-chain or the fourth and fifth fraction of an α2-chain. Kang (1972) has in fact, shown that a cross-link does occur between α1CB1 (containing the N-terminal telopeptide) and α1CB6. There are in addition to the lysine residues, approximately one-third as many hydroxylysine residues grouped specifically in the C-terminal half of the molecule. All these can theoretically provide the other half of linkages originating in the 9α1 or 6α2 allysine residues, since in addition to linkages in those CNBr fractions listed above, which can only form *intra*-microfibrillar bonds, there are also linkages which provide lateral *inter*-microfibrillar bonds throughout the length of the tropocollagen molecule.

The nature of the intramolecular bonds. Two δ-amino adipic acid semi-aldehydes (allysine residues originating in pairs of α-chains) can interact by aldol consensation with the formation of an unsaturated aldehyde (Fig. 40). Bailey and Robins (1972) who first suggested that this structure might provide the cross-linkage between individual α-chains in the tropocollagen molecule were also of the opinion that it might in some as yet unexplained fashion act as the precursor of more complex *inter*molecular cross-linkages (see below).

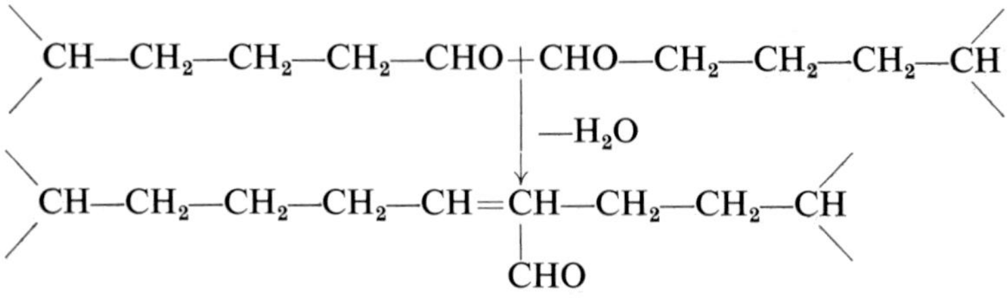

$$\diagdown CH-CH_2-CH_2-CH_2-CHO + CHO-CH_2-CH_2-CH_2-CH \diagup$$

$$-H_2O$$

$$\diagdown CH-CH_2-CH_2-CH_2-CH=CH-CH_2-CH_2-CH \diagup$$

$$CHO$$

FIG. 40. The production of allysine aldol by the condensation of two molecules of allysine.

The intermolecular bond. Aldehydes produced by the oxidative deamination of lysine or hydroxylysine residues, can not only interact with other aldehydes, but also with amino groups which are terminal to the side chains of lysine residues which have not suffered oxidation.

Theoretically four different Schiff's bases or aldimines can be produced from the various selections of lysine, hydroxylysine, allysine and hydroxyallysine (Fig. 41) with no hydroxyl group, one hydroxyl group in position 1, or 2 hydroxyl groups in both these carbon atoms.

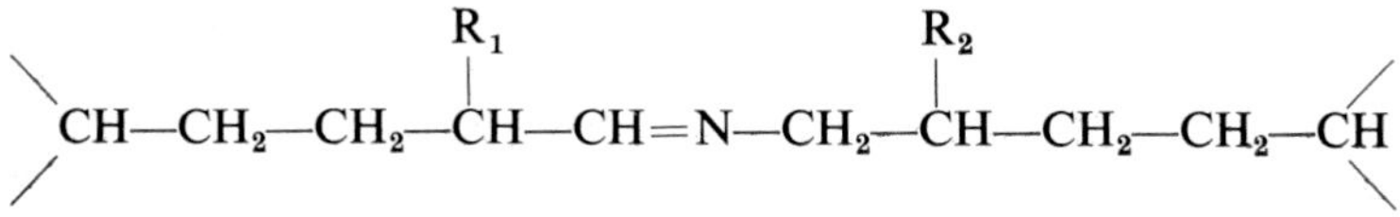

$$\diagdown CH-CH_2-CH_2-\overset{R_1}{\underset{|}{CH}}-CH=N-CH_2-\overset{R_2}{\underset{|}{CH}}-CH_2-CH_2-CH \diagup$$

FIG. 41. Theoretically possible Schiff's bases which can be formed from various lysine derivatives. R_1 can represent either H or OH and R_2 also H or OH. Four combinations of these are possible.

The first confirmation of the existence of labile Schiff's bases of this type was obtained by Bailey and Peach (1968) who isolated N-ε-(5-amino-5-carboxypentyl)-hydroxylysine, commonly known as hydroxynorleucine, from an acid hydrolysate of borohydride reduced collagen. They suggested that this compound is derived from the Schiff's base, dehydrohydroxylysinonorleucine, which will have been formed in the native protein by the condensation of the aldehyde group of an allysine residue and the amino group of a residue of hydroxylysine.

Lysinonorleucine and dihydroxynorleucine are both minor components of reduced mature skin collagen, but the latter occurs as a derivative of one of the major cross-linking species in the collagen of tendon, cartilage and bone.

Davis and Bailey (1971) have shown that the naturally occurring precursor of this more complex cross-link, also known as syndesine, is derived by Schiff's base formation between a molecule of hydroxyallysine and a molecule of hydroxylysine. As a cross-link it is more stable than might be expected of an aldimine and Robbins and Bailey (1973) have ascribed this phenomenon to the possibility of spontaneous Amadori re-arrangement to give a more stable Ketonic structure:

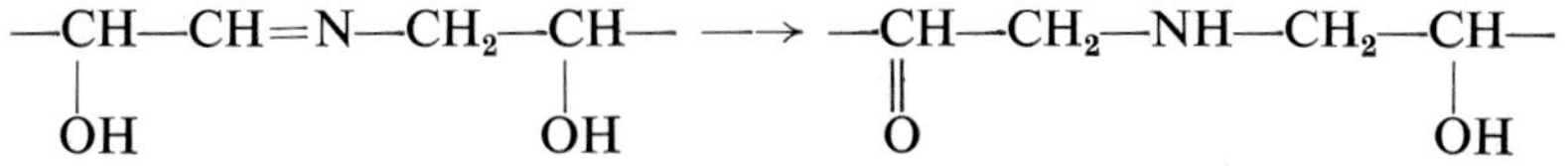

$$-CH-CH=N-CH_2-CH- \longrightarrow -CH-CH_2-NH-CH_2-CH-$$
$$\quad\ |\qquad\qquad\qquad\ \ | \qquad\qquad\quad\ \ |\qquad\qquad\qquad\qquad\ \ |$$
$$\quad\ OH\qquad\qquad\qquad OH\qquad\qquad\quad O\qquad\qquad\qquad\qquad OH$$

Another cross-link has been identified by Bailey and Lister (1968); and Franzblau *et al.* (1970). It is eluted from ion exchange columns immediately after histidine, and was originally given the name Fraction C or the post-histidine peak. Tanzer *et al.* (1973) using a mass spectrographic and NMR approach have suggested that it is synthesised by the Michael addition of a histidine residue through the imino group of its imidazole ring to the intra-molecular allysine-aldol linkage and the subsequent addition of a hydroxy-lysine residue to this complex via Schiff's base formation (Fig. 42).

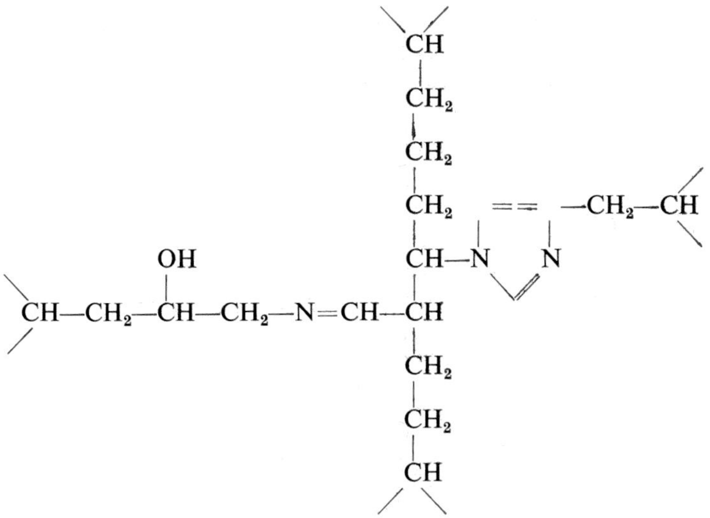

FIG. 42. Possible structure for the cross-linking component "C".

The *in vivo* existence of a compound of this exact structure has been questioned, and it has been suggested that the final complex, as isolated, may be an artefact, since it cannot be hydrogenated with borohydride without the release of a concomitant amount of the aldol condensation product. However, some complex linkage of this type must exist in the native tissue, since the appearance of Fraction C is accompanied by a reduction in the *intra*molecular aldol linkage, and treatment with phosphate buffer results in the release of a large amount of this same aldol.

Tissue specificity. The various cross-linkages are distributed in varying amounts throughout collagens of different tissues and species (Table 3). Some tissues contain only one species of cross-link, some two and a number all three. It is possible that the incidence of these different cross-links may be dependent on the nature of the individual α-chains. Bailey and Robins (1973), for instance, record that tissues in which the collagen consists of three α1-chains, such as cartilage, all possess dehydro-dihydroxylysinonorleucine as their major cross-linking structure. The reverse is, however, not the case; this particular linkage also being present in uterine collagen, although this protein consists of both α1- and α2-chains. Where α2-chains do occur in a species of collagen there is evidence for them to be preferentially cross-linked at the expense of the α1-chains, leading to a predominance of β_{12} dimers and α1 monomers when the denatured soluble collagen is fractionated on acrylamide gel. An alternative explanation to that involving the sub-unit composition of the collagen could be that the nature of the cross-links is dependent on the degree of hydroxylation of the lysine in the N-terminal telopeptide.

TABLE 3. Distribution of types of cross-links among various tissues.

Cross-link type	Tissue
Dehydro-hydroxylysinonorleucine and Fraction C	Dermis
Dehydro-dihydroxylysinonorleucine, dehydro-hydroxylysinonorleucine and Fraction C	Tendon
Dehydro-dihydroxylysinonorleucine	Bone and cartilage

Dehydro-dihydroxylysinonorleucine occurs in the main in those tissues which are least soluble, and it may be that the possibility of an Amadori re-arrangement to give the more stable keto-structure as mentioned above, is responsible for this. Tendons and other soft collagenous tissues contain, in addition to dehydro-diOH-L.N.L. the other more labile forms of aldimine linkage, and now that the nature of these various bonds is appreciated, their existence can be seen as confirmation of a phenomenon first reported by Veis (1965), namely that collagen contains both labile and resistant forms of co-valent linkage.

Fraction C is virtually absent from bone, cartilage and uterine collagens, indicating that *inter*molecular cross-linkages are produced early in the development of these tissues at the expense of the *intra*molecular linkages which might have subsequently developed into Fraction C linkages. This may indicate that these tissues require stable *inter*molecular links soon after synthesis to produce the insoluble collagen required for their specialised functions. Bone and cartilage have early supportive roles, whilst the uterine tissue must mature rapidly because of its ephemeral nature.

Age variations in cross-linkages. Robins *et al.* (1973) have studied the relative changes in the types of cross-linkage occurring in bovine skin collagen over an age range from foetal to fully adult (7 years). Dehydrodihydroxylysinonorleucine, which is the major cross-linkage present in foetal skin falls to about one-third its initial level by birth, and has disappeared almost entirely by 6 months of age. The presence of this cross-linkage, which in tissues from adult organisms is associated with a high degree of stability, confers the unexpected degree of insolubility which is typical of foetal skin collagen. Within a few months of birth this highly resistant cross-link is replaced by dehydrohydroxylysinonorleucine and Fraction C both of which rise during the first 18 months of life, until together they account for nearly 90% of the total number of cross-links. The remaining 10% consists mainly of partially characterised glycosylamines. This form of cross-link increases steadily with age after birth, and from 18 months of age onwards, does so at the expense of the dehydrohydroxylsinonorleucine and Fraction C linkages. At 6 years of age over 60% of the total cross-linkages are glycosylamine in nature. Similar observations have been made for human skin collagen, where the peak concentrations of the two cross-links dehydrohydroxylysinonorleucine and Fraction C occur at 17–20 years of age (Bailey and Shimokomaki, 1971). Robert *et al.* (1971) have reported on the ratio of cross-linking amino acids in rat tail tendon to the lysine content over the age range 1 to 24 months. Over this period the high-voltage electrophorectic method which they employed for the separation of the amino acids did not permit any significant changes in the amount of cross-linking amino acids relative to lysine to be recorded. If anything the total cross-link content appears to tend towards a reduction (22.5%) during the first 10 months, followed by a return almost to the preweaning level during the next 14.

It is well-known that the collagen which is laid down in the tissues of young animals is being continuously metabolised to permit the remodelling of the developing tissues (p. 150) and these observations of Bailey and his colleagues demonstrate that different forms of collagen are synthesised during foetal, infantile and pre-mature growth. Fraction C, whether it contains the histidine grouping which renders it capable of cross-linking four α-chains or not (p. 91) is definitely synthesised by development from the intramolecular aldol bond to produce a more complex intermolecular linkage. The collagen which is synthesised during the later weeks of pregnancy and in increasing amounts thereafter, during periods of maximum growth up to maturity, would first appear to be cross-linked within the tropocollagen molecules, which are subsequently bound together to form the elongated microfibrillar structures associated with mature collagen. The changes which take place when growth ceases after maturity, appear to be dependent on the formation of bonds between the microfibrils and glycoproteins.

Jackson and Bentley (1968) have suggested that post-maturity collagen is bound to glycoproteins and to glycosaminoglycans and Bailey's observations would appear to indicate that these linkages, which appear after borohydride reduction, in the form of hexitol-lysine residues (Robins *et al.*, 1973) continue to be produced in increasing amounts after all the possible *intra-* and *inter-* molecule bonds have been formed.

Heikkinen (1969) has reported that the number of cross-linkages in the collagen of rat tail tendon increases from one link for every half million daltons to one for every 50 000 daltons as the animal ages from 3 to 100 weeks. Considering intermolecular linkages only, this amounts to an increase in cross-linkages from six between every five pairs of tropocollagen molecules to twelve between every pair. This constitutes a considerable increase in the number of points at which the α-chains of the individual tropocollagen molecules are closely bound together, and can easily explain the observations of Heikkinen (1968); Cadavid *et al.* (1963); Mills and Bavetta (1966); Nimni *et al.* (1966) and Wirtschafter and Bentley (1962) who have reported on average an 88% reduction in the amount of collagen which is extractable from rat skin by neutral sodium chloride solution during the first 12 months of life.

Non-lysine based linkages. Other linkages in addition to the aldols and aldimines discussed above, have over the years been suggested as stabilising factors in the collagen molecule. Few, however, have been fully substantiated, but their presence in specific sites must not be ruled out completely. Notable among such hypothetical linkages have been the following. Ester linkages: originally believed to exist between possible sub-subunits (Gallop *et al.*, 1959); such subdivision has since been proved to be incorrect. Biphenyl linkages derived from tyrosine: these may be associated with pigmentation and the fluorescence of the protein (see section on elastin cross-links) (Harding, 1965; Joseph and Gowri, 1970). γ-Glutamyl and α-amino peptide linkages (Mechanic and Levy, 1959): the formation of pseudopeptide linkages between these two amino acids is most probably an artefact brought about during hydrolysis of the protein. Aromatic side chain substitutions of phenylalanine and tyrosine (Cooper and Davidson, 1965) have not been substantiated.

Elastin

Elastin content of ageing tissues

Human vascular system. Since 1938 a variety of methods has been employed for the estimation of the elastin content of connective tissues. Many of them have been used to determine the way in which the elastin content of these tissues change with age. The number of different results which have been reported are almost as numerous as the different methods employed, and this is especially apparent in the case of determinations of elastin in the aortic wall. Vascular tissue from the larger arteries of young subjects consists of two main scleroproteins, collagen and elastin together with a small amount of muscle protein, and of proteins associated with polysaccharide, in the ground substance. This protein mass accounts for between 90 and 95 % of the total dry weight of the tissue, and the collagen and elastin together make up nearly 60 % of this, the muscle proteins actin and myosin constituting the majority of the remainder. In the smaller arteries and arterioles the proportion of muscle proteins is increased at the expense of collagen and elastin. In the large arteries of older subjects collagen and elastin are joined by pseudoelastin (p. 112), and the properties of this third protein are such that it is included together with the collagen fraction in certain methods of tissue analysis, and with the elastin in others. In some methods, however, the pseudoelastin appears to be divided between these two major protein fractions.

The methods which have been employed for the estimation of elastin depend either on the removal of collagen and the soluble proteins, to leave a solid residue, or on the specific dissolution of the elastin using the pancreatic enzyme, elastase.

Methods for the removal of collagen and soluble proteins include autoclaving with water (Stein and Miller, 1938; Lowry *et al.*, 1941; Miller *et al.*, 1952; Miller *et al.*, 1953; Neuman and Logan, 1950; Harkness *et al.*, 1957) boiling with dilute alkali, (Lansing *et al.*, 1950; McGavack and Kao, 1960; Scarselli, 1960) with dilute acetic acid, (Balo and Banga, 1949; Hall and Gardiner, 1955) with formic acid, (Lloyd and Garrod, 1946; Ayer *et al.*, 1958) with urea, (Hall, 1951; Bowen, 1953) extraction with guanidine chloride, (Miller and Fullmer, 1966; Ross and Bornstein, 1969) and treatment with cyanogenbromide, (Rasmussen *et al.*, 1975). A number of groups of workers have employed two or more of these relatively drastic methods for the removal of both collagen and soluble proteins (Buddecke, 1958; Walford *et al.*, 1959) while various groups have compared a number of methods (Walford *et al.*, 1959; Banga, 1969; Hall, 1968a; Sandberg, 1975). Fitzpatrick and Hospelhorn (1960) and Serafini-Fracassini *et al.* (1975) were not confident that these drastic procedures left the elastin residue in an entirely undamaged state. Certainly the observations of Hall (1951, 1955) had shown that elastin could be completely dissolved by boiling 8M urea and by boiling 0.1N NaOH, and the latter was confirmed at a later date by Labella and Vivian (1967). Fitzpatrick and Hospelhorn, therefore, attempted the purification of elastin by alternate digestion with crystalline trypsin and collagenase until no further protein was liberated. The residue apparently consisted of elastic fibres in an undamaged state, but the amino acid analysis of this residue (Table 4) differed markedly from that of classical elastin (Partridge and Davis, 1955; Petruschka and Sandberg, 1968) and may therefore, have contained other protein entities than elastin itself. Sandberg (1975) suggested that where enzymic purification is employed, inhibitors of non-specific proteolytic enzymes should also be present to protect the elastin molecule.

TABLE 4. Amino acid composition of various elastin preparations.*

	A	B	C	D	E	F
Hydroxyproline	15	11	11	11	8	10
Aspartic acid	9	3	7	11	5	4
Threonine	7	12	15	14	8	14
Serine	8	9	11	11	9	12
Glumatic acid	21	19	20	27	16	17
Proline	94	126	126	125	108	104
Glycine	329	362	362	255	327	326
Alanine	233	247	240	236	220	230
Cysteine	0	0	0	0	0	0
Valine	125	159	156	155	154	132
Methionine	0	0	1	3	0	0
Isoleucine	20	27	27	26	24	16
Leucine	57	63	65	68	65	45
Tyrosine	17	21	22	22	8	16
Phenylalanine	32	25	25	24	30	26
Hydroxylysine	0	0	0	0	0	0
Ornithine	1	7	3	2	2	1
Lysine	8	9	6	6	8	43
Arginine	7	8	8	10	4	4
Histidine	1	trace	1	2	trace	0
Desmosine and Isodesmosine	16	3	12	9	16	0
Lysinonorleucine						0

* Residues/1000. A, Elastin from adult pig aorta; B, Elastin from foetal pig aorta; C, Elastin from human adult aorta (20 yrs); D, Elastin from elderly human aorta (85 yrs); E, Elastin from ox ligamentum nuchae; F, Elastin from copper deficient pig aorta.

The values reported by various groups of workers for the elastin content of human aortas of various ages depend therefore, on the method employed, but as is demonstrated in the section on amino acid analyses (p. 106) the firmness with which elastin is combined or at least associated with pseudoelastin is itself age dependent. Therefore, those workers who employed methods which were based on the removal of collagen and other soluble proteins but who used solvents which were incapable of disrupting the linkages which bound elastin and pseudoelastin together, would record elastin levels which were higher than they should be, due to the retention within the elastin preparation of a fraction originally derived from collagen. Thus Lansing *et al.* (1950a) observed a fall in the elastin content of aortic media from 48% at the end of the second decade to 41–43% at the beginning of the sixth decade, but noted that the level rose again slightly (to 44%) during the seventh and eighth decades, only to fall again by the time the ninth decade was attained. These variations in elastin content are in close agreement with the observation of Labella *et al.* (1966) who reported the existence of a protein with an abnormal amino acid analysis in the aortas of a group aged 51–60 years (p. 111). Kraemer and Miller (1953) by reason of their choice of age groups were not in a position to observe any alteration in elastin content, the level for the 0–50 year old group ranging from 30.8–41.7. The increased scatter of values for their older group may indicate that the younger members of this group (aged 50–60) might here again provide higher values than those of more advanced age. Any assessment of those changes in elastin content which are due to age alone is rendered difficult by the fact that arteriosclerotic changes are more prevalent in the aged than in the young. Buddecke (1958) examined the aortas of 50 subjects ranging in age from 4 to 80 years, but because he divided his subjects by degree of arteriosclerosis, obtained three groups, the ages of which overlapped to a considerable degree. The aortas of his youngest group (4–39 years) were completely free of arteriosclerotic plaques and had elastin contents with a mean value of 28.6%. The second group which had a medium degree of arteriosclerosis and ranged in age from 33 to 79, although including those subjects who might be expected on the basis of Labella's observation to carry in their aortas a mass of firmly bound pseudoelastin, had a mean value for elastin content of 22.9%. The heavily arteriosclerotic group (53–80) which again might include among its younger members an appreciable number of those with firmly bound pseudoelastin had an even lower elastin content (16.8%). Buddecke employed a mixture of methods for the purification of elastin, including cold 0.5N NaOH for 15 hours to remove the glycosaminoglycans, autoclaving with water to remove the collagen, and a final purification of the residual elastin with 0.1N NaOH. It is possible that the preliminary treatment with relatively concentrated cold alkali, followed by a high temperature at a neutral pH results in the removal of some stabilising factor thus rendering the linkages between elastin and pseudoelastin labile to hot dilute alkali.

It appears likely that the elastin content of aorta rises over the first 20 years of life (Walford *et al.*, 1959) and falls thereafter. (Fitzpatrick and Hospelhorn, 1965) 1–15 years, 40–48; 15–35 years, 34; 45–55 years, 33; 55–58 years, 26 and 61–79 years, 18–39. Over a period which may be considered as "late middle age" the total elastin and pseudoelastin level increases, but again over this period and during subsequent years the effect of an increasing degree of arteriosclerosis is to lower the elastin level by a considerable amount.

Methods of analysis in which the elastin is dissolved by pancreatic elastase, either directly from whole tissue or after partial purification (Scarselli, 1959, 1960) have been employed by a variety of workers. Scarselli stained whole elastic tissue sections or sections which had been treated with 0.1N NaOH at 25 °C for 18 h with acid orecin. Studies of the absorption spectrum of the dye alone and when combined with the digestion products of elastin demonstrated a shift in the optimum absorption from 574 nm to 589 nm, thus indicating the formation of a co-valent linkage between the dye and the protein. More drastic hydrolysis freed the whole of the dye which could then be shown to have been combined with the protein to the extent of 1.256 %. The release of these dyed digestion products after elastolysis could be used as an estimate of the elastin content. Salvini (1960) and Scarselli *et al.* (1960) using this method reported falling levels of elastin in aortic wall with increasing age, but the two sets of workers reported markedly different values for the elastin contents of the individual age groups (Table 5). A possible explanation of this has recently been provided by Hall *et al.* (1973).

TABLE 5. Protein fractions in aortic media of human subjects of varying ages extracted by elastase and remaining after exhaustive extraction with boiling decinormal alkali. (mg/g)

Age	Elastase extract	Alkali residue	Pseudoelastin
2 months	339	214	125
21 months	376	218	158
47 years	362	224	138
75 years	461	220	241

Hall (1971) and Tesal (1971) showed that there are a number of forms of elastase secreted by the pancreas (p. 156). The enzyme is normally extracted from pancreatic tissue at pH 4.7 (Balo and Banga, 1950; Hall and Czerkawski, 1959). Extraction at other pH values, however, also permits the removal of active enzyme from pancreatic tissue. The enzyme which is mainly extractable between pH 4.5 and 6.5 is soluble in buffer or salt solutions of ionic strength 0.1–0.5, but precipitates on dialysis, whereas the major part of the enzyme preferentially extractable at pH 1.4 is fully soluble in water. This soluble enzyme is of higher molecular weight and contains a relatively high concentration of calcium (up to 2.1 %), whereas the other water insoluble species contains relatively little calcium (0.02–0.04). Tesal (1971) and Hall *et al.* (1973) have shown that pure preparations of a calcium-rich and a calcium-poor species of elastase can be isolated from these crude extracts of pancreatic tissue by electrofocusing in ampholine columns, and that the crude extracts contain respectively 4 parts of the calcium-rich species to one of the calcium-poor form and 8 parts of the calcium-poor form to one of the calcium-rich.

Theoretically the enzyme-substrate complexes formed by the interaction of the calcium-rich enzyme with those regions of the substrate which contain free carboxyl and hydroxyl groups and those which are formed by the interaction of the calcium-poor enzyme with calcium cross-linkages in the substrate, should be identical, but Hall and El-Ridi (1976b) using calculations based on the graphical method of Eisenthal and Cornish-Bowden (1974) have shown that the Michaelis-Menten constants are different when the two enzymes are allowed to act on a substrate which may be assumed to contain both calcium free and cross-linked regions. The mean value for the Michaelis constant for reaction involving the calcium-poor enzyme is 90 ± 20 mg/ml, whereas that for the calcium-rich enzyme is 30 ± 2 mg/ml. These differences must indicate that the primary and secondary structure of the substrate affects the reaction either from a steric point of view (Hoare, 1972), or because the localisation of other charged groups close to the reactive centre alters the ease with which enzyme and substrate can approach one another, or conversely the ease with which the enzyme can separate from the products of reaction.

These two enzyme preparations have been used to study the age changes in the elastin and co-ordinately bound calcium content of human aorta (Hall *et al.*, 1973). The intima, the inner layers of the media, the middle region of the media and the adventitia from non-atherosclerotic areas of aorta from human subjects aged 21 to 75 years were gently freed of lipid, soluble collagen and other soluble material and treated separately with the two elastase preparations described above. The reactions were carried out at pH 8.7 (the water insoluble enzyme) and pH 7.8 (the soluble preparation) at concentrations relative to the weight of air dried tissue of 0.05 and 0.1 % respectively. The susceptibility of the media rose from 68.2 % at 21 years to 89.1 % at 75 years of age in the case of the insoluble, calcium-poor enzyme, and from 45.3 to 78.1 over the same age range for the calcium-rich enzyme. The intima, inner media and adventitia were also more susceptible to both enzymes in elderly subjects. If, however, the ratios of the susceptibilities are calculated for elastin preparations from the various tissues at each age (Table 6) it can be seen that whereas the relative susceptibility of elastin from the mid-portion of the media falls with age, that of elastin in the immediately sub-intimal region and even more so in the intima itself, rises with age. From this it can be deduced that the relative amounts of substrate which are specifically digested by the calcium-poor enzyme increase in the intima, and other immediately peri-luminar regions, whereas the substrate decreases in concentration relative to that component which is specific for the calcium-rich enzyme in those regions of the wall which are more distant from the lumen. Thus the amount of co-ordinately bound elastin increases in the intima with increasing age at the expense of non-cross-linked elastin, and *vice versa* in the middle and outer layers of the media. The use of quantitative elastolysis to measure the elastin content of vascular tissue will therefore depend on four factors:

1. The calcium content of the tissue – hence the degree of arteriosclerosis.
2. The relative amounts of the two enzymes present in the elastase prepara-tion employed.
3. The proportions of media and intima in the tissue sample examined.
4. Age.

and attempts to utilise this method to correlate quantitative assessments of elastin to the fourth of these factors may be markedly affected by any or all of the other three.

TABLE 6. Ratios of the susceptibilities of various sections of normal human aorta at different ages to digestion by the two forms of elastase (E) and (ECa) expressed as a percentage. (From Hall *et al.*, 1973.)

Tissue	21 yrs	47 yrs	75 yrs
Intima	67.3	92.4	105.4
Inner media	92.4	99.7	108.6
Media	150.5	145.8	114.1

The apparent increase in elastin content in the 63–88 year age group re-ported by Scarselli *et al.* (1960) may be due to the fact that elastin from this group which is classified by the authors as being a group with a high incidence of advanced arteriosclerosis, and hence most probably severely calcified, has been digested by an enzyme preparation containing a higher proportion of the calcium-poor form of elastase. Banga (1969) employed elastolysis for the estima-tion of the collagen content of aortic tissue, using the enzyme to disolve both the elastin and any denatured collagen present (cf. Banga, 1953; Hall *et al.*, 1953) and reported appreciable but variable amounts (between 2 and 48%) of so-called "other components"; in other words those which could neither be classed as elastin because they remained after alkali treatment or as collagen because they remained after elastolysis. In two of the eighteen samples on which she reported, the sum of "elastin" and "collagen" were respectively 16 and 27% greater than the weight of tissue examined. This must imply the existence of material which is not soluble following treatment with elastase, but which remains undissolved in alkali. Its existence in 11 % of the samples throws doubt on the values obtained for the others. Using straight elastolysis of unstained tissue, Banga found much larger values for elastin content ranging from 47 to 82 % but if the tissue was stained with orcein first, and then subjected to elastolysis, the range of values was reduced to 45–74 %. A proportion of the stained tissue could be released following alkali treatment thus reducing the "true" elastin levels to the range 25–45 %, well within the range covered by other workers' results. The upper values of this range together with a value of 40 % were surprisingly enough recorded for two patients aged 91 and 86 respectively.

Balo and Banga (1955) also studied the velocity of elastolysis in young and old aortas, and showed that the older elastins were more rapidly dissolved than the younger ones. Labella (1962) on the other hand reported exactly opposite findings. Banga (1966) suggested that Labella's observations were erroneous because of a faulty turbidimetric technique. She suggested that the high calcium phosphate content of the "elastase resistant" old elastin preparations, maintained the high turbidity of the reaction mixture even after the elastin protein had been dissolved. Most of this calcium component is the EDTA extractable material reported by Yu and Blumenthal (1958) and bears no direct relationship to the co-ordinately bound form of the metal, the presence of which in addition to the extractable calcium salt would increase the susceptibility of the substrate to attack by the water insoluble, calcium-poor form of the enzyme. If, however, the water soluble form of the enzyme is employed, the results reported by Labella would be obtained whatever the method used to follow the course of the reaction. A further difficulty in assessing the changing rate of elastolysis and using this to indicate alterations in the structure of elastin or its content in elastic tissues, is due to the fact that pseudoelastin appears in increasing amounts in aortic tissues from elderly subjects and this has long been known to be susceptible to attack by elastase, (Hall et al., 1953; Banga, 1953) and if it has not been removed from the tissue before the elastolytic reaction is allowed to proceed, its degradation products will be included together with the soluble elastin in any measurement of elastase activity.

Vascular tissues of animals other than man. Estimations of the elastin content of aortic tissue from animals other than man, although quite widespread, has not been applied to age studies to any great extent. Harkness et al. (1957) studied the carotid, subclavian and innominate arteries in the dog, together with different regions of the ascending thoracic and abdominal aorta to determine the levels of total solid, collagen and elastin. They reported that the differences which could be observed between the various forms of vascular tissue, namely a variation from an essentially elastin-rich region near to the heart, to collagen-rich tissues, elsewhere, were much more significant than any changes which could be unequivocally attributed to age. They based their conclusion on the observation that the pattern of protein distribution was equally apparent in the new-born and the adult dog. However, the intra-thoracic vessel did suffer a loss of elastin of from 70 to 60 % with approaching adulthood, and the changes in the peripheral vessels were even greater, falling from 60 to 25 % during maturation.

In the rat the elastin content of the aorta rises rapidly over the first 5 months and then the rate of increase falls with age. The most significant observation (Hall and Loeven, 1975) is that the elastin content of rat aorta is greater at all ages up to 24 months in the male than in the female. This is in close agreement with the observation that the amount of elastase available in the male system, by synthesis in the pancreas, is at all times higher in the case of the female rat. If, as is believed, (Balo and Banga, 1949; Hall and Loeven, 1975) elastase is responsible for the maintenance of a given level of elastic tissue in the body (cf. p. 153) then the higher level in the female could be related to the main-tenance of the lower elastin content which is observed. Twenty-four months may not represent an appreciable proportion of the total life span of the rat, and this rise in elastin may merely correspond to the rise in the elastin level of human aortic tissue reported by Walford et al., 1959, during the attainment of maturity or conversely it might indicate the existence of a completely different mode of elastin metabolism in the rat. Cleary and McCloskey (1962), investigated the distribution of elastin in the arteries of rabbits, and its varia-tion with age. The rapid increase in elastin at the expense of collagen which is apparent in human aortas during the first years of life was not seen in the rabbit. However, measurement of the total weights of both collagen and elas-tin in the growing rabbit demonstrated that both fibrous proteins were being laid down in increasing amounts as the vessel grows. They suggested that the hydrostatic pressure in the arteries of the upper trunk and neck is less in the case of animals such as the dog, the cat, the rat, the goat and the rabbit, than in the case of upright animals such as man and the kangaroo. It is possible that the rapid increase in the elastic elements of the artery wall are directly related to this variation in pressure. Hall and Slater (1973) have suggested that at later ages the effect of recurrent stress such as that associated with the pulse may induce the degradation of the collagen with the association of its degrada-tion products with glycosaminoglycans derived from the surrounding ground substance. Viola et al. (1960) demonstrated a progressive decline to 16 % of the original value in the rate of uptake of ^{14}C-glycine by rats of increasing age. Similarly, Kao et al. (1960) studying the incorporation of ^{14}C-lysine observed a significantly higher rate of uptake by the aortas of 5-week old rats than by those of 8-month or 2-year old animals, whilst Walford et al. (1964) again studying glycine uptake suggested that any alteration in aortic elastin which may occur with age is not accompanied by its resorption and reconstitution. In general, therefore, it may be concluded that the rate of elastin synthesis falls off with age, and if the elastin of the aortic wall is degraded as age progresses, no replacement ensues. This is in agreement with the observations of Hall and Loeven (1975), and may indicate that at advanced age the elastin content may fall.

Skin. McGavack and Kao (1960) reported that the elastin content of rat skin decreases markedly with age (from approximately 1.13% to 0.42% between 20 and 5000 days of age). In contrast, Hult and Goltz (1965) observed no age changes in the elastin content of human skin using a micro densitometric assessment of orcein stained sections. Although such methods of assessment are subject to considerable error (Hall, 1971) due to their dependence on the angle at which the section through the skin is cut, Varadi and Hall (1965) also observed little marked change in elastin levels in the skin over the age range 6–40. The values obtained however, depend so much on the history of the skin sample concerned, and on the method employed for analysis that the results reported by each group of workers have to be considered separately.

The study of the ageing of dermal tissue has been bedevilled over the years by the fact that it has proved very difficult to differentiate between those changes in skin which were directly age related, and those which were due to exposure to actinic radiation. Histologists such as Kissmeyer and With (1922); Ejiri (1936, 1937) and Tattersall and Savile (1950) reported that the typical petichiae distributed beneath the surface of the skin of the face, forearms and backs of the hands of elderly people were accompanied by an increase in the amount of elastica-staining material in the immediately sub-epidermal third of the dermis. Hill and Montgomery (1940) observed that these histological changes were observable only on those surfaces of the body which were exposed to sunlight, the inner aspect of the forearm of an elderly subject showing normal histology (Fig. 18) whilst a section from the outer aspect appeared clogged with elastica-staining material. Lansing (1954a, b) suggested that these fibrous masses were true elastin, since they stained typically with elastica stains such as resorcinolfushsin and Verhoef's reagent, and were digested with elastase, but this had already been queried by Tunbridge *et al.* (1952) and doubts were later cast on this hypothesis by Hall *et al.* (1955). Tunbridge *et al.* (1952) demonstrated that the elastosis which had been reported by earlier workers was apparent rather than real, being due to the presence in the dermis of large masses of degraded collagen fibres (Fig. 19). They showed that the appearance in the electron microscope and the staining properties of the elastica-staining material in the senile exposed dermis resembled that of the degraded collagen which resulted from short term treatment of native collagen fibres, with pepsin.

This controversy was continued for a number of years, Findlay (1954) joining Lansing in defining the material present in senile skin as elastin on the basis of its elastase susceptibility, while Braun-Falco and Salfeld (1956, 1957a, b) used a variety of methods for the study of the dermis, and on the basis of these, also identified the material present in senile conditions as true elastin. The false premise on which at least the deductions from elastase susceptibility observations were based had already been demonstrated. Banga (1953) and Hall *et al.* (1953), had shown that collagen denatured by a variety of methods becomes susceptible to attack by elastase, hence the existence of material which can be dissolved by elastase cannot be taken as unequivocal evidence that it is true elastin.

Gillman *et al.* (1955a, b) approaching the question of pathological dermal tissue solely from a histological point of view, observed "basophilic degeneration" of collagen fibres in sections stained with haematoxylin, and showed

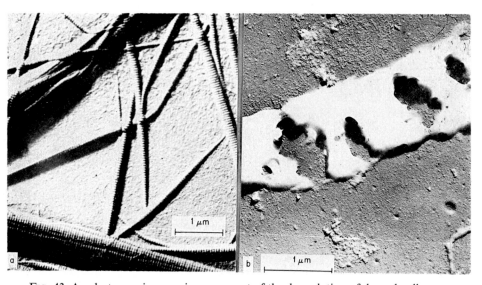

Fig. 43. An electron microscopic assessment of the degradation of dermal collagens of varying age by clostridial collagenase. (a), Production of tactoid forms from individual microfibrils. (b), Production of electron dense pseudoelastin.

that the areas which stained in this fashion were co-terminous with areas which stained with elastica stains in senile skin. Hence it could be deduced that not all material which stains as elastic tissue can be classified as true elastin. This observation demonstrated the close parallelism which exists between elastica-staining material in the dermis and in the aorta.

Keech (1954a) had shown that collagen fibres from the skins of subjects of increasing age showed marked differences in their mode of susceptibility to *clostridial* collagenase, as visualised in the electron microscope. Thus young fibres were virtually completely taken into solution (Fig. 43) as at a slower rate were fibres from elderly subjects. At all stages during digestion the residue could be transformed into gelatin by boiling. Fibres from young adult subjects on the other hand, even after prolonged treatment with collagenase did not dissolve completely, but left behind an amorphous residue which was resistant to boiling water, merely consolidating into an electron-dense mass. Banga *et al.* (1956) prepared a similar material, to which they gave the name metacollagen by treating collagen with various lyotropic substances such as potassium thiocyanate, potassium iodide and sodium perchlorate. They showed that this material had many properties similar to those of elastin, namely: elasticity, staining, lack of birefringence and acid swelling and digestibility by proteolytic enzymes notably, elastase.

This derived tissue component which has been named "pseudoelastin" (Hall, 1964) "metacollagen" (Banga, 1966) or "elastolytically degraded collagen" (Gillman, *et al.*, 1955a, b) "collastin" (Unna, 1896; Loewi *et al.*, 1960) and "old elastin" (Lansing *et al.*, 1951), appears to occur with increasing age in a number of connective tissues, especially in those which already contain elastin. The properties and amino acid analysis, however, appear to vary from tissue to tissue. Slater and Hall (1973) have devised a method which is capable of differentiating between true elastin and pseudoelastin, especially in the dermis. Pseudoelastin is represented by that fraction of the tissue which can be extracted by elastase, but which does not remain undissolved after treatment with alkali. Two determinations, therefore; a gravimetric assessment of true elastin by extraction with alkali, and a colorimetric estimation of all the material extractable with elastase – true elastin and pseudoelastin – provide the data from which the pseudoelastin content can be determined. In abdominal skin there is a 25 % drop in true elastin over the first six decades, followed by a slight rise (not more than 10 % on average) during the remainder of the life span. The pseudoelastin content, starting at a lower level also falls, but only during the first two decades, and then increases three-fold during the rest of life (Fig. 44). This observation is in contrast to those made by Smith *et al.* (1962a) in which all the changes reported in skin are attributed to the effect of ultra-violet irradiation. This phenomenon does have an effect, however, on exposed sites, Slater and Hall (1973) observed nearly twice as much pseudoelastin in the cheek, forehead and forearm skin of subjects aged 56–68 years as in their abdominal dermis. It would appear therefore, that although the effects of ageing alone are apparent in skin which remains covered throughout life, the more profound alterations observable in the exposed skin of elderly subjects is a composite effect made up partly of age-mediated factors and partly of other factors due to actinic activity.

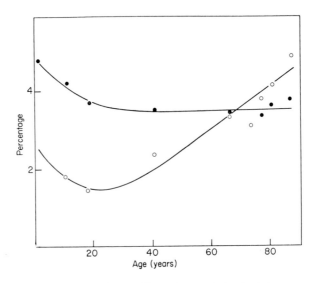

FIG. 44. Age changes in the elastin (●) and pseudoelastin (O) content of human abdominal dermis.

The composition of elastins of varying age

Amino acids. The first recorded analytical data for the amino acid composition of hydrolysates of elastin, which might remotely lay claim to being representative of the whole protein, were those provided by Stein and Miller (1938). Prior to this time methods of amino acid analysis were so complicated that no single worker was likely to be able to provide values for more than one or two amino acids, and even these analyses required such large amounts of protein as starting material, that the number of tissues which could be studied, was limited. In effect only ligamentum nuchae, containing as it does approximately 80% elastin was capable of analysis by these earlier methods of analysis. Elastins from tissues such as lung, vascular wall and dermis, consisting in the main of collagen, could in general only be studied as pooled samples, and then usually only from animals such as the ox from which large amounts could be obtained. It was not until more sensitive methods of analysis were available that tissues from smaller animals or from human subjects, and hence specifically from subjects of different ages, could be examined. The development of methods of microbiological assay (Lansing *et al.*, 1951), paper chromatography (Hall, 1951b, 1955) and column chromatography (Neuman, 1949; Neuman and Logan, 1950; Partridge and Davis, 1955; Fitz-patrick and Hospelhorn, 1960; Serafini-Fracassini and Tristram, 1966; Grant, 1966) permitted increasingly accurate analyses to be made from ever smaller amounts of tissue.

The first direct evidence that elastic fibres suffer changes in their amino acid composition with increasing age was provided by Lansing and his colleagues (Lansing *et al.*, 1948; Lansing *et al.*, 1950b, 1951). They observed that elastin from aorta, after being freed from collagen by repeated treatment with boiling dilute alkali can be separated into light and heavy fractions when finely ground and centrifuged in sucrose solution (s.g., 1.30). The heavy fraction contains high concentrations of calcium (cf. p. 39) whereas the light one is essentially calcium free. Most of the material present in the four young tissues (15–20 years of age) studied by Lansing remained suspended in the sucrose solution, whereas the majority of the older tissue (6 subjects aged 55–75) precipitated. Amino acid analyses of these two fractions (Lansing *et al.*, 1951) demonstrated marked changes in the levels of certain amino acids. Table 7 records mean values and standard deviations for the amino acids: aspartic and glutamic acids, leucine, isoleucine and valine and for the imino acid, proline. The table also contains figures for the means and standard deviations for the amounts of the same amino acids in pulmonary arteries

TABLE 7. Comparison of partial amino acid analyses (g/100g protein of elastin preparations from the aortas and pulmonary arteries of two age groups of human subjects. Group A (15–20 years) gave so-called "light" preparations of elastin in both tissues, Group B, (55–75 years) gave "heavy" elastin when prepared from the aorta. (Lansing *et al.*, 1951.)

	Aorta			Pulmonary artery		
	Group A	Group B	p.	Group A	Group B	p.
Aspartic acid	0.31 ±0.06	1.07 ±0.41	0.005	0.67 ±0.014	0.54 ±0.12	N.S.
Glutamic acid	1.51 ±0.16	2.48 ±0.36	0.001	1.91 ±0.105	1.57 ±0.25	N.S.
Glycine	26.5 ±0.05	24.3 ±1.1	0.005	30.85 ±0.64	33.10 ±1.98	N.S.
Leucine	4.8 ±0.2	4.8 ±0.1	N.S.	4.82 ±0.20	4.74 ±0.30	N.S.
Isoleucine	2.3 ±0.07	2.4 ±0.12	N.S.	2.26 ±0.03	2.30 ±0.23	N.S.
Proline	11.15 ±0.26	10.2 ±0.72	N.S.	10.96 ±0.46	10.8 ±1.4	N.S.
Valine	13.0 ±0.55	11.5 ±0.46	0.005	12.9 ±1.0	12.9 ±0.71	N.S.

N.S. = No significant difference.

from smaller groups of young and old subjects. The elastin preparations from these pulmonary arteries were shown to consist almost entirely of the "light" fraction after sucrose centrifugation. From Table 7 it can be seen that "heavy" elastin samples from elderly aortas contain significantly greater amounts of the acidic amino acids, glutamic and aspartic acids, than do samples from young tissues. The glycine and valine contents of the elastin on the other hand fall significantly with age, but the levels of leucine, isoleucine and proline remain roughly constant; the slight variations with age not being significant. On the basis of these observations Lansing and his colleagues suggested that the amino acid composition of elastin in the aorta changes with age, no significant changes being observable in the elastin fraction from the wall of the pulmonary artery. However, they could not justify the assumption that this shift in amino acid distribution represented an actual change in the amino acid analysis of a single protein already laid down in the tissue. The general theory of protein synthesis which has developed since 1951 is also in conflict with such a possibility, since there is little likelihood of amino acids already incorporated into a protein being removed and replaced by others. A more likely explanation would appear to involve the laying down alongside the existing elastin of another protein with properties which are so similar, that it segregates along with elastin in the course of purification, but which differs from classical elastin in its amino acid analysis to such an extent as to provide analytical values for individual amino acids in the mixture which are similar to those reported by Lansing. Lansing and his colleagues proposed that this second protein should be regarded as a new form of elastin but Hall and his colleagues (Burton *et al.*, 1955; Hall *et al.*, 1955; Hall, 1957, 1959, 1968a) basing their observations equally on chemical and morphological studies (p. 112) of ageing elastic tissue put forward the suggestion that this second elastic protein is in fact derived from pre-formed collagen. Because of its properties (p. 105) they named it pseudoelastin; a title which had first been proposed by Gilman *et al.* (1955a, b) on purely tinctorial grounds. Hall (1951, 1955) and Bowen (1953) observed that elastic tissue – especially that present in the aortic wall – could all be dissolved in boiling 8M urea solution, if the ratio of solution to solid was maintained above 20:1. This treatment is a development of the method employed by Stein and Miller (1938) for the removal of collagen from elastic tissue, and Hall suggested that the retention by these workers of an elastin residue at the end of their treatment was due to the fact that the liquor-solid ratio which they employed was relatively low. Using a semi quantitative method, based on the visual assessment of paper chromatographs, Hall showed that the collagen fraction was removed first: the residue gradually becoming essentially free of hydroxyproline. The last fraction which dissolved, after 90 h boiling, had an amino acid analysis which was characteristic of normal young elastin from ligamentum nuchae (Partridge and Davis, 1955), but between the collagen and the elastin, a fraction was dissolved having an amino acid analysis which appeared to be part way between that of collagen and that of elastin. In later experiments (Hall, 1968a) in which the amino acid content of elastin from the aortas of cattle aged 2, 4, 6 and 7 years was measured following hydrolysis and fractionation on a column of spherical ion exchange resin, it was observed that seven amino acids in the elastin from the 4-year old cattle were increased in concentration (hydroxyproline, aspartic acid, threonine, serine, glutamic acid, tyrosine and phenylalanine) when compared with the composition of the elastin from either the 2- or 7-year old aorta. On the other hand five acids (namely: glycine, proline, alanine, leucine and isoleucine) were present in lower concentration (Table 8). Labella *et al.* (1966)

TABLE 8. Comparison of the amino acid analysis of elastin preparations from the aortas of 4-year old cattle with those of similar preparations obtained from 2- and 7-year old beasts. The figures indicate the ratios of the concentrations of the individual acids. (Hall, 1971).

Amino acids with raised conc. in 4-year old cattle		Amino acids with lowered conc. in 4-year old cattle	
Hydroxyproline	4	Alanine	0.8
Aspartic acid	4	Isoleucine	0.5
Threonine	3	Leucine	0.9
Serine	2	Lysine	0.1
Tyrosine	2	Valine	0.9
Arginine	5		
Histidine	5		

Changes in other amino acids were not significant.

similarly compared the amino acid compositions of different age groups of human subjects and showed comparable peak levels of certain amino acids in elastin from aortas of the 51–60-year old group (Fig. 45). Although 4-year old cattle would not appear to correlate directly, as far as biological age is concerned, with a group of human subjects in their sixth decade, the same phenomenon appears to occur in both species. At some point in "middle life", a second protein, fails to separate from the elastin as the purification process proceeds. It is quite acceptable that this protein may be completely absent from the younger tissues, and may subsequently develop with age, but its apparent disappearance from the tissues of the most elderly group requires more explicit explanation. There are two possible reasons why two proteins will segregate together in the same fraction during a purification procedure aimed at the preparation of one of them. The two may have such a similar physical and chemical composition that they cannot be separated by the

method being employed or they may actually form a complex with one another. The profound difference in amino acid analysis which must exist between the two proteins under consideration if the average composition of the
mixture is to differ so markedly from that of elastin, must render it infinitely
more susceptible to hydration and hence make it more soluble, than the
hydrophobic apolar structure of classical elastin. It may, therefore, be assumed

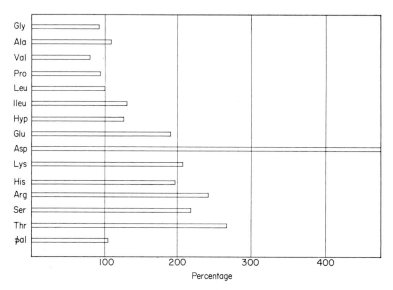

FIG. 45. The percentage proportion by which each amino acid in aortic elastin from
the 51–60-year old group differs from the mean values of analyses for elastin from
11–20, 31–40 and 81–90-year old groups.

that the two proteins interact with one another to form what may be regarded
as a "middle-aged elastin complex". The nature and strength of the bonds can
be deduced from the type of reagent which brings about the disruption of the
complex, notably 8M urea which is a well proved reagent for the fission of
hydrogen bonds. Middle age is not, however, the only period during which
complex formation occurs between elastin and some other protein fraction.
Foetal elastin (Cleary et al., 1966; Labella and Vivian, 1967; Hall, 1968) also
has a very unclassical amino acid analysis (Table 9) (cf. p. 96).

The observation that collagen, pseudoelastin and elastin can be separated
by serial extraction with 8M urea solution is further borne out by the findings of
Serafini-Fracassini and Tristram (1966) who used more sophisticated methods
for the purification of aortic elastin, removing calcium and collagen simultaneously by exhaustive extraction with ethylene diamine tetra acetic acid.

They reported closer similarity between analyses of elastins from normal adult (20–30 years) and old (60–70 years) aortas, than was claimed by Lansing and his colleagues or by Labella *et al.* (1966). Although their "old" group was of a different age span to that which has been referred to above as "middle aged" by Labella *et al.*, it was still many years below the "old" group as defined by this pair of workers (81–90 years). It would appear that the mode of purification is of considerable importance in determining whether pseudo-elastin can be separated from true elastin. Dilute acetic acid (Hall, 1955) or dilute alkali (Lansing *et al.*, 1951) alone, are incapable of severing the bonds which hold pseudoelastin and elastin together. Urea (Hall, 1955), formic acid (Ayer *et al.*, 1958) and ethylene diamine tetra acetic acid followed by dilute alkali (Serafini-Fracassini and Tristram, 1966) are all capable of breaking the bonds between elastin and pseudoelastin, dissolving the latter and leaving a residue with the classical amino acid analysis.

TABLE 9. Amino acid composition of foetal* bovine aortic elastin compared with that of normal adult elastin, (residues/1000). (Steven and Jackson, 1967.)

Amino acid	Foetal	Adult
Hydroxyproline	12.4	11.4
Aspartic acid	5.0	8.2
Threonine	4.6	7.1
Serine	6.6	9.0
Glutamic acid	16.3	14.0
Proline	104.0	97.5
Glycine	325.2	325.0
Alanine	224.7	232.3
Valine	143.5	145.2
Methionine	trace	trace
Leucine	26.6	26.5
Isoleucine	64.4	64.2
Tyrosine	8.7	13.1
Phenylalanine	25.6	30.3
Isodesmosine	4.1	4.4
Desmosine	5.9	5.7
Lysinonorleucine	2.0	1.3
Ornithine	1.6	1.4
Lysine	5.5	6.8
Histidine	0.9	trace
Arginine	5.2	5.0

* The foetal age was assessed by size as 30 in. from crown to rump.

Glycoprotein components of elastin. Various workers have identified a microfibrillar component in foetal elastic tissue (Ross and Bornstein, 1969; Robert *et al.*, 1971), which represents about 8% of the total tissue mass. As the fibres mature the relative proportions of these non-elastin glycoproteins and elastin itself change as elastin is synthesised, probably using the microfibrillar component in much the same fashion that the registration peptides of pro-collagen are used. A comparison of the amino acid analyses of these two proteins indicates that they are very similar, lacking hydroxyproline, hydroxylysine and the desmosines but containing a high content of cystine.

In collagen the registration peptides constitute a part of the procollagen molecule, whereas in elastin the same alignment function would appear to be provided by a separate molecule. Hoffman et al. (1974) have shown that the microfibrils have no role to play in the physical stability of the molecule, but during elastogenesis they delineate the dimensions of the growing fibre. At full maturity the microfibrils are completely embedded in amorphous elastin protein, and with normal staining techniques are no longer visible in the electron microscope. Cliff (1971), however, has shown that prolonged periods of staining with osmium tetroxide can reveal an underlying microfibrillar structure even in mature tissue.

In advanced age there is evidence for an increased synthesis of glycoprotein following the reduced synthesis which can be observed during all earlier periods following the cessation of foetal development. This age-glycoprotein is very similar in composition to the microfibrils, but whether it is laid down in the same form is not yet certain. It may be closely related to the pseudo-elastin, the origin and composition of which is discussed below.

Pseudoelastin

Chemical composition. Tunbridge et al. (1950, 1952) observed collagen degradation products in the exposed dermis of elderly subjects in areas which had previously been shown (Kissmeyer and With, 1922; Ejiri, 1936, 1937) to stain heavily with elastica stains. In place of the fine strands of elastin or the clear cross-striated collagen which is present in normal unexposed young skin, these areas contain broken and bent collagen fibres covered with an amor-phous layer. This material is elastase susceptible (Lansing et al., 1953) but no longer susceptible to collagenase (Loewi et al., 1960). Hall (1968a) suggested that this material which was in fact partially degraded collagen, was similar to the substance which Gillman et al. (1955a, b) had identified in certain patho-logical skin conditions by histochemical means, and possibly also to the entities which Unna (1896) had reported in skin and which on the basis of the relation-ship of their staining properties to those of elastin on the one hand and col-lagen on the other, had called elacin, collastin and collacin.

Tunbridge et al. (1952) observed that collagenous tissue treated for short periods of time with pepsin assumed the staining properties of elastin, and became partially degraded and covered with an amorphous coat when viewed in the electron microscope. Subsequent studies demonstrated that a number of different methods could be employed for the conversion of collagen into a material with many of the properties of collagen, (Burton *et al.*, 1955; Hall and Tunbridge, 1957; Hall, 1956; Keech *et al.*, 1956) and it was observed that during such treatment portions of the collagen molecule were removed.

Lansing *et al.* (1950a, b, 1951) were the first to suggest that the composition of elastin altered with age, but notwithstanding the observations of Hall and Labella's group, this suggestion has been repeated more recently by Ebel *et al.* (1970); Kramsch *et al.* (1971) and Kramsch and Hollander (1973) as being applicable to elastin from the region of the atherosclerotic plaques. Although ageing may occur without any atherosclerotic involvement, the opposite would not appear to be the case, and it may well be that the changes that occur in atherosclerosis bear no relationship to the changes which occur in ageing. On the other hand the linkages which bind together pseudoelastin and elastin in middle-aged tissue and which are not susceptible to attack by dilute acid or alkali, but which can be broken by urea, may be replaced in the atherosclerotic plaque by co-valent linkages which are resistant even to urea. Whether the pseudoelastin is bound to elastin by urea-labile hydrogen bonds or by more stable linkages, its presence in association with elastin in middle-aged non-atherosclerotic tissue, but not in samples from more elderly subjects, poses an interesting question. How does relatively insoluble and unreactive pseudoelastin once it has been synthesised in middle age disappear from older tissues? Hall (1973a) has suggested that pseudoelastin is produced by the action of tissue collagenases on collagen fibres which are partially cross-linked (Fig. 46). Young uncross-linked collagen will suffer complete degradation under the action of such degradative enzymes. Old heavily cross-linked collagen will also be broken down; not the same low molecular weight products but to small cross-linked entities by enzymes which are able to penetrate between the cross-links which hold the molecule rigid and prevent its collapse. Partially cross-linked molecules will tend to collapse once a limited number of main chain peptide linkages are broken, producing an amorphous mass such as that observed by Keech (1955). This material could have properties which are characteristic of pseudoelastin, namely: loss of organisation, altered tinctorial properties, increased elasticity and altered solubility both in dilute acid and alkalis and under the action of collagenase. The observations of Keech (1954b, 1955) and Hall (1956, 1957) appeared to indicate that pseudoelastin is completely resistant to collagenase. This is certainly true of *clostridial* collagenase, but may not necessarily hold for those collagenases which originate in the homologous connective tissue itself. Hence, if the increasing cross-linkage of aged collagen militates against the further production of pseudoelastin and that which is produced in middle age is itself slowly destroyed, the lower levels of this protein which are apparent in extreme age can be explained. In the atherosclerotic plaque, the combination of lipid with the pseudoelastin, may not only render it more firmly bound, but may also make it more resistant to further degradation by collagenase. This is obviously an aspect of artery wall metabolism which warrants further study.

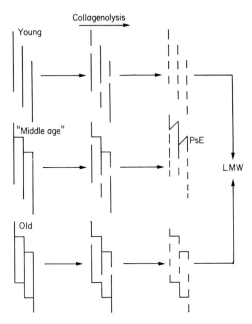

Fig. 46. Diagrammatic representation of the degradation of collagens of varying degrees of cross-linkage to indicate the possible route whereby pseudoelastin may be produced preferentially from the sparsely cross-linked "middle-aged" collagen.

Pseudoelastin in skin. Chemical and biochemical methods have proved of inestimable value in the assessment of the relative amounts of collagen, elastin and pseudoelastin in dermis. Varadi and Hall (1965) demonstrated that the true elastin content of dermis is between 2.77 and 3.17%. They employed hot alkali extraction for the removal of associated proteins and thus assured the complete removal of all nonelastin protein. It has, however, been shown recently (p. 95) that less drastic methods of extraction may provide an elastin preparation which is more closely related to its physiological state. Prolonged alkali treatment may result in the removal of a small amount of the elastin molecule itself. Slater and Hall (1973) suggest, however, that there may be an intermediate period during which the amino acid composition of the extracted tissue remains constant. This residue may be regarded as being true elastin freed from collagen, and from any collagen degradation products which are recognised as pseudoelastin.

Exhaustive treatment with elastase not only dissolves the true elastin component, but also all that portion of the collagen originally present, which has been converted by age-dependent processes to pseudoelastin. It is one of the fundamental characteristics of elastase that it is without effect on native undenatured collagen, and hence the only difference between the amount of elastin remaining in the residue from alkali-treated tissue, and the total protein dissolved by elastase is the pseudoelastin component. This is of course, only true when all other soluble components, such as immature collagen and ground substance have been previously removed by extraction with neutral salt solutions. Otherwise they would be included in the elastase extractable material.

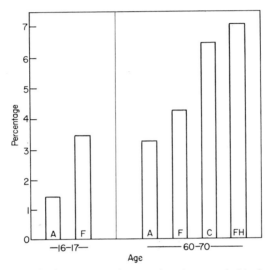

FIG. 47. The pseudoelastin content of covered and exposed skin from two different age groups. A, abdominal; F, forearm (outer aspect); C, cheek; FH, forehead.

The amounts of pseudoelastin determined in this fashion which are present in abdominal skin from subjects ranging in age from 2 months to 85 years (Slater and Hall, 1973) show a 50% fall during infancy and adolescence followed by a four-fold increase over the next seventy years. Although the elastin content of the tissue also falls to begin with, thereafter it remains roughly constant at this reduced level (Fig. 44). Even young abdominal elastin contains a finite amount of pseudoelastin but the four-fold increase between 11 and 85 years of age represents a considerable increase which can only be ascribed to the ageing process, since in this instance the skin being from the abdomen has not been subjected to ultra-violet irradiation. Slater and Hall (1973) also report actinic changes, however, in pseudoelastin content demonstrating the presence of up to twice as much pseudoelastin in skin from the cheek and the forehead as from the abdomen in the same age group. These observations are at variance with those of Lansing (1955) who suggested that the apparent elastosis in senile skin is in fact a true elastosis, and of Smith *et al.* (1962) who not only claimed to have confirmed Lansing's observation, but also suggested that the changes as observed were in no way age mediated but were solely due to ultra-violet irradiation.

The amino acid analyses of elastin prepared by alkali extraction from elderly unexposed abdominal skin and from elderly cheek or from skin from the exposed aspect of the forearm differ from one another and also from classical analyses for ligamentum nuchae elastin (Table 4). The tyrosine level for instance is three times greater in the forearm skin elastin than in the classical analysis and there are other smaller variations.

It would appear, therefore, that the use of elastase for the isolation of elastin from tissues which may also contain collagen degradation products is not justifiable. Nor can treatment with alkali remove the whole of the non-elastin protein from a tissue, since although alkali can remove all the pseudo-elastin from elderly unexposed tissue, at least a portion of the pseudoelastin which exists in irradiated skin is resistant to alkaline extraction. Hall (1973b) has also observed different pseudoelastins in diseased states. The pseudo-elastin present in the skin of subjects with pseudoxanthoma elasticum not only appears to be different from that present in senile skin (Tunbridge *et al.*, 1952) but is less susceptible to elastase.

Hall (1970b) has shown that repeated cycles of mechanical stress and relaxation exerted during and following precipitation of collagen from solution will bring about changes in solubility and enzymic susceptibility. Stretched collagen fibres become increasingly insoluble in dilute acid, and decreasingly susceptible to attack by collagenase, while demonstrating increasing susceptibility to elastase. Skin is under constant flexion and relaxation during life, and it may be that part at least of the change in properties of collagen as it is converted to pseudoelastin is brought about as the result of the physical trauma experienced during life.

Examination of a single case of cutis laxa (Hall, 1969b) has led Hall to postulate that the production of pseudoelastin is a normal concomitant of the ageing process. The symptoms of cutis laxa in this particular subject developed progressively from the neck and face downward across the chest and abdomen during a six year period in which the appearance of the skin of the face altered dramatically so as to give the impression of a 20 to 30 year increase in age. Postmortem abdominal skin samples from this subject therefore, were of greatly differing apparent age to those obtained from the neck. The elastin content of these two samples were only slightly different, whereas the pseudo-elastin content increased 40-fold with apparent age, i.e. between the abdomen and the neck.

This was probably a unique occurrence, but the apparent age gradient across the torso permitted longitudinal ageing studies to be made on a single subject, thus eliminating any individual variation which may render cross-sectional studies on ageing less convincing.

Pseudoelastin in the large blood vessels. Hall and Slater (1973) have shown that the pseudoelastin content of the media of the ascending aorta of human subjects remains essentially constant up to 47 years of age, and then increases in amount considerably at greater ages. They were able to demonstrate that the pseudoelastin component of the aorta becomes increasingly associated with polysaccharide with increasing age, the ratio of polysaccharide to protein (μg/mg) rising from 29.1 at 21 years of age to 46.4 at 75. Similar elution profiles for both polysaccharide and protein on Sephadex G100, indicate that the protein and polysaccharide are co-valently bound to one another not just loosely associated in the tissue. Similarly the artificial production of a pseudoelastin-like substance by repeated stretching and relaxation (Hall, 1970b) results in the retention of polysaccharide. These recent observations confirm the claim (Hall, 1951, 1955) that pseudoelastin is present in increasing amounts in ageing aorta. Nearly 20% more protein is extracted during the first three 24 h periods of treatment with boiling 8M urea solution from a 67-year old aorta than from a 20-year old one (Hall, 1964). This is accompanied by a 14% decrease in the amount of collagen which is extractable by dilute acetic acid (thus indicating a possible origin for the pseudoelastin), and by the extraction of a 33% greater amount of polysaccharide.

It may be assumed therefore, that the degradation of collagen in both the dermis and the aorta results in the production of a product which reacts with polysaccharide with the production of material which has many of the properties of elastin. Some of this material becomes closely associated with the native elastin of these tissues, and is isolated along with elastin in many of the preparative procedures for this protein.

Cellulose-containing fibres. Hass (1943) reported the presence in connective tissue of structures which he termed *anistropic splints* in addition to the usually identifiable collagenous and elastic fibrous elements. In 1958 Hall and his co-workers (Hall *et al.*, 1958) isolated highly anisotropic structures from human dermis, and later from aorta (Hall *et al.*, 1960) following the removal of ground substance, collagen and elastin by exhaustive treatment with salt solutions, collagenase and elastase (Fig. 48). These structures contain a high concentration of carbohydrate and a smaller protein moiety. Certain of the fibres can be seen to consist of two structural components, a central isotropic core surrounded by a series of highly anisotropic helixes winding in opposite senses round the core. In 89% of the fibres the angle of the helices is 72° to the axis of the fibre. In those fibres in which the core is completely covered,

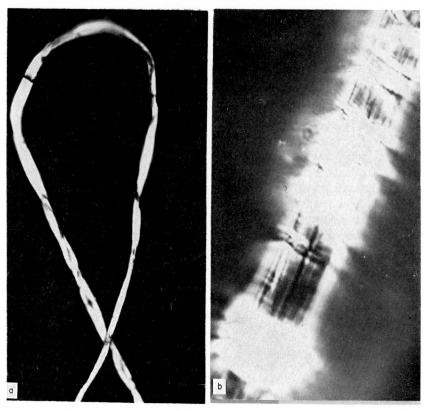

FIG. 48. Cellulose from human dermis, viewed in plane polarised light. (a) Fibre showing marked anisotropy at all modes of alignment to the plane of polarisation (×200); (b) Fibre partly stripped of outer anisotropic coat showing two opposed helically wound anisotropic elements (×1 000).

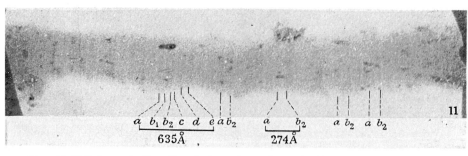

FIG. 49. Cellulose micelles aligned along the surface of collagen fibril covering the a, b_1 and b_2 striations.

the sheath retains its anisotropy at all settings of the polarisers. This must indicate that the helical structure consists of a series of individually anistropic mycelles lying in close association with collagen fibrils and invariably overlapping the a, b_1 and b_2 bands (Fig. 49).

Both chemically and by X-ray diffraction criteria the polysaccharide component of the fibres was identified as cellulose (Hall *et al.*, 1958, 1960; Hall and Saxl, 1960, 1961). The protein core which is not susceptible to attack by collagenase or elastase, has an amino acid analysis which lies midway between collagen and elastin and is therefore similar to the group of collagen-derived proteins to which the name pseudoelastin has been given.

The degradation of collagen under conditions which have been shown to result in the production of pseudoelastin (Burton, *et al.*, 1955; Hall *et al.*, 1955) results in the formation not only of fibrous masses which stain like elastin, but also in the production of highly anisotropic fibres (Fig. 50). It has been demonstrated (Hall and Slater, 1973, cf. p. 115) that both naturally occurring pseudoelastin from elderly subjects and similar material prepared by cyclical stretching and relaxation results in the close binding of protein and polysaccharide. The artificial fibres may not consist of protein-cellulose complexes, but it appears that where the precursors of the cellulose mycelles are available for attachment to the protein derived by the degradation of collagen, the anisotropic fibres identified in various connective tissues can be produced.

An examination of the anisotropic fibre content of connective tissues from subjects of a variety of ages proved that at all ages above 20 a limited number of fibres were visible. The small but finite number of fibres apparent in all adult tissues could not be proved to increase with age, but below maturity they could only be observed sporadically. The largest number was observed in the skin of a subject with Scleredema of Buschke, showing that the formation of cellulose containing fibres can be induced not only by age, but also by disease processes.

Hitherto cellulose has only been demonstrated in the animal kingdom in the silkworm (Shimizu, 1955; Buonocore, 1958) and in the test of the tunicates (Mark and von Susich, 1924). Hall and Saxl (1961) compared the appearance and chemical composition of human cellulose fibres and the material from the test of the tunicates – tunicin, and showed that the protein core to which the cellulose is attached is pseudoelastin-like in both cases. Tunicin only appears in the sessile, adult stage of the organism being completely absent from the free-living notochord-bearing larval stage. It has been suggested that it is from the larval state of an organism of this type that the vertebrates have developed, presumably among other things by the repression of those genes which control the metamorphosis to the adult state and the synthesis of cellulose. It is possible that the appearance of cellulose in human and other

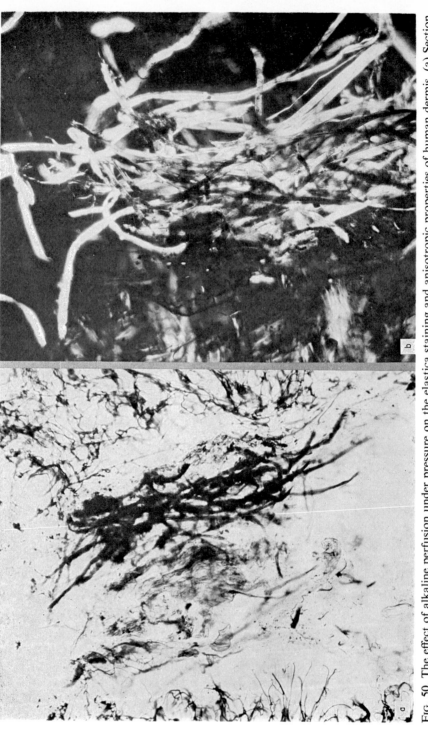

FIG. 50. The effect of alkaline perfusion under pressure on the elastica staining and anisotropic properties of human dermis. (a) Section through a sheet of human dermis prefused for 72 h with alkaline buffer, then fixed and stained with Weigert's elastica stain. The mass of elastica-staining fibrils lines the area of final rupture. (b) The area of rupture viewed between cross Nichol prisms. (×250)

animal connective tissues represents the age-mediated de-repression of these gene loci.

Cross-linkages in elastin

Lysine-derived linkages. Partridge *et al.* (1964) and Thomas *et al.* (1963) isolated two new polyfunctional amino acids from partial hydrolysates of elastin. These were subsequently shown to consist of substituted quaternary salts of pyridine, derived by the condensation of three allysine residues and one lysine residue.

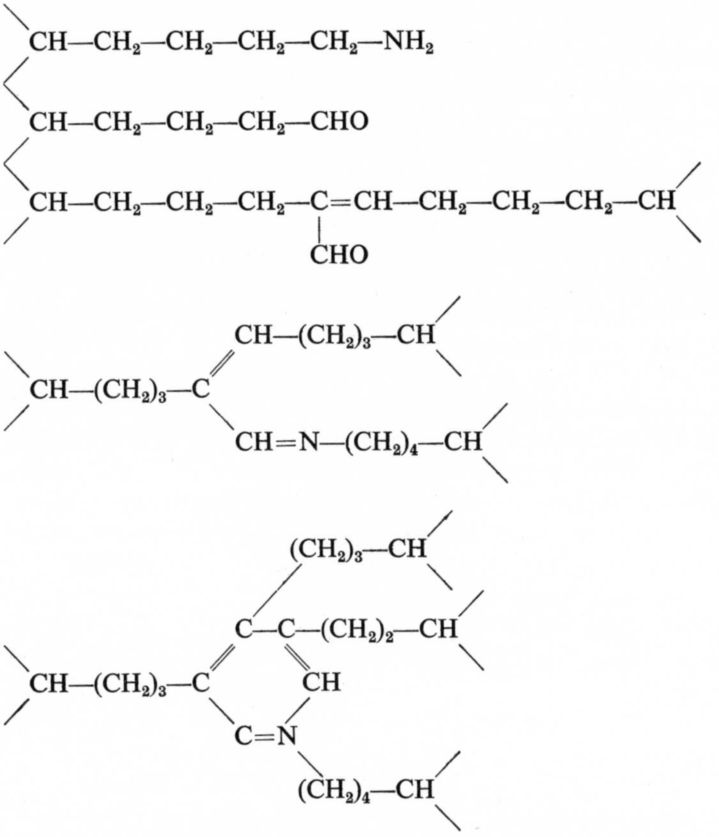

$$\text{CH—CH}_2\text{—CH}_2\text{—CH}_2\text{—CH}_2\text{—NH}_2 \qquad \text{Lysine}$$

$$\text{CH—CH}_2\text{—CH}_2\text{—CH}_2\text{—CHO} \qquad \text{I}$$

$$\text{CH—CH}_2\text{—CH}_2\text{—CH}_2\text{—C=CH—CH}_2\text{—CH}_2\text{—CH}_2\text{—CH} \qquad \text{II}$$
$$\underset{\text{CHO}}{|}$$

III

$$\text{CH—(CH}_2)_3\text{—CH}$$
$$\text{CH—(CH}_2)_3\text{—C}$$
$$\text{CH=N—(CH}_2)_4\text{—CH}$$

IV

$$\text{(CH}_2)_3\text{—CH}$$
$$\text{C—C—(CH}_2)_2\text{—CH}$$
$$\text{CH—(CH}_2)_3\text{—C} \qquad \text{CH}$$
$$\text{C=N}$$
$$\text{(CH}_2)_4\text{—CH}$$

FIG. 51. Intermediate structures in the production of elastin cross-links from lysine, I allysine, II allysine aldol, III merodesmosine, IV desmosine.

They and subsequent workers, suggested that the symmetrically substituted pyridine-desmosine could be derived from one allysine aldol molecule (Fig. 51, II) and an intact lysine, by Schiff's base formation between the mid-chain aldehyde group of II and the amino group of the lysine, followed by the addition of a third allysine molecule to the product of this reaction (III) across the conjugated double bond system to give an N, 3,4,5 tetra substituted pyridine (IV) desmosine. The asymmetrical iso-desmosine could arise from a different form of interaction between the final allysine residue and intermediate III to give an N, 3,5,6 tetra substituted ring. Each of these structures can link four adjacent polypeptide chains by virtue of the fact that the lysine residues from which they are synthesised may originate in four separate polypeptide chains, but Foster *et al.* (1973) and Gerber and Anwar (1974) have suggested that the roots of the desmosine linkages may be located in pairs in two chains rather than singly in four.

Over the past ten years each of the intermediate stages in the synthetic scheme outlined in Fig. 52, or their reduction products, have been identified in small amounts in native elastin, or following borohydride reduction. Franzblau *et al.* (1965) first isolated lysinonorleucine, whose structure indicated that it had probably been synthesised by the reduction of the Schiff's base formed between one residue of allysine and one intact lysine residue (Fig. 53). Lent and Fránzblau (1967) later identified the un-reduced Schiff's base itself in elastin, thus confirming this synthetic route for the production of lysinonorleucine. Miller and Fullmer (1966) also identified allysine and what was most probably the aldol condensation product of two such molecules – allysine aldol, (Fig. 51, II) and finally Starcher, *et al.* (1967) and Paz *et al.* (1971a, b) isolated small amounts of a new trifunctional amino acid – merodesmosine – from reduced elastin, indicating that the non-reduced form of this complex amino acid (Fig. 51, III) might well exist in native elastin. Piez (1968) draws attention to the fact that the proposed synthetic route outlined above, whereby the desmosines are produced, only represents one of a number of possible

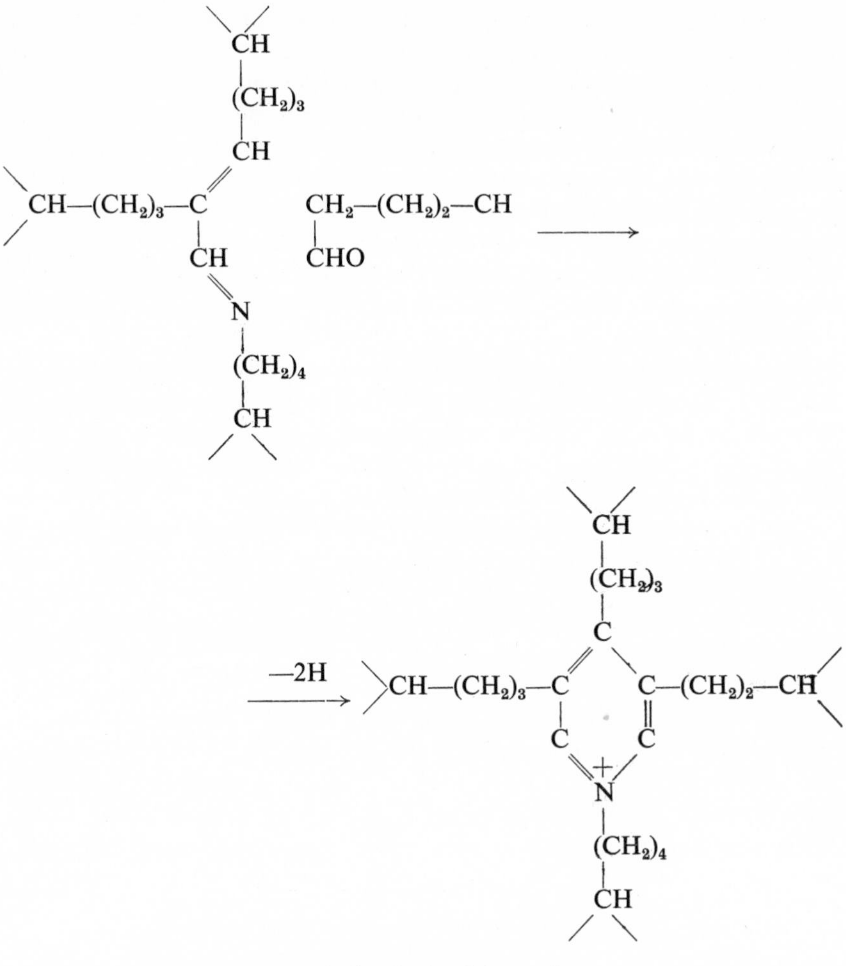

FIG. 52. Synthesis of desmosine.

reaction mechanisms, but the identification of certain of the intermediates in tissue hydrolysates led initially to the conclusion that it may well represent the correct pathway. More recent observations by Franzblau (1971) and Francis *et al.* (1973), have, however, provided evidence for another possible mechanism for desmosine production, based on a Michael reaction between the aldol condensation product formed from two allysine molecules which occurs in large amounts in foetal tissue and a third allylysine residue to give a trilysyl dialdehyde. Such a complex could then interact with an intact lysine residue to complete the desmosine ring. This pathway differs, from the one outlined above in that the Schiff's base reaction which introduces the nitrogen atom which ultimately becomes the quaternary nitrogen of the desmosine ring, occurs as the last step in the synthesis rather than at an intermediate stage.

Another possibility which has much to recommend it, especially if the linkages are visualised as joining pairs rather than four separate chains requires the preliminary production of an *intra*-chain allysine aldol on one polypeptide and an *intra*-chain dehydrolysinonorleucine on another. These two may then interact by oxidative condensation to produce the desmosines.

$$CH—CH_2—CH_2—CH_2—CHO + H_2N—CH_2—CH_2—CH_2—CH_2—CH$$

$$\Big| \quad —H_2O$$

$$CH—CH_2—CH_2—CH_2—CH{=}N—CH_2—CH_2—CH_2—CH_2—CH$$

$$\Big| \quad +2H$$

$$CH—CH_2—CH_2—CH_2—CH_2—NH—CH_2—CH_2—CH_2—CH_2—CH$$

Fig. 53. Synthesis of lysinonorleucine.

Studies of the peptides containing the cross-linkages have been reported by Foster *et al.* (1973, 1974) and Gerber and Anwar (1974). In those studies the sequence of amino acids around the desmosine, isodesmosine and lysinonorleucine cross-links have been identified, and it has been shown that the lysine residues which form the bases of these linkages are invariably surrounded by alanine residues. Where there is evidence for the desmosines linking pairs rather than groups of four polypeptide chains, the pairs of lysine residues from which the linkages stem are separated by two or three alanine residues (Fig. 54).

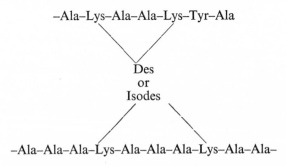

Fig. 54. The relationship of the desmosine linkages to alanine residues in a pair of adjacent elastin chains.

Partridge pointed out that the intermediate aldols and Schiff's bases required for these synthetic pathways are labile, and the early linkage of two or three elastin chains is of necessity a reversible process. He suggests that the non-permanence of these bonds will permit the remodelling of elastic tissues before the protein chains are irrevocably bound together by stable desmosine and isodesmosine linkages.

The lysine-derived cross-linkages of elastin have one fundamental difference from those of collagen, in that they may occur in their reduced forms – lysinonorleucine, hydroxylysinonorleucine and di- and tetrahydrodesmosine (Paz *et al.*, 1974) – as well as in the original unsaturated state, whereas the cross-linkages of collagen have only been identified in the reduced form after the tissue has been treated with borohydride. Allysine aldol which has been identified as the *intra*molecular cross-link in collagen has also been reported as a linkage joining two chains in elastin (Lent *et al.*, 1969) from studies involving the administration of ^{14}C-lysine to chick embryo cultures. In exactly the same way that the aldol can both form linkages in its own right and also act as a precursor for the Fraction C linkage in collagen (p. 91) it would appear likely that in elastin it also has a dual role. There are 4 to 5 allysine aldol per 1000 amino acid residues, indicating that it exists as an integral cross-linking element in elastin, but it can also take part in the formation of the desmosines (Fig. 55).

2 lysines → 2 allysines—*intra*-chain allysine aldol   (A)

2 lysine → 1 lysine+1 allysine → *intra*-chain Schiff's Base   (B)

A+B → *inter*-chain desmosine

FIG. 55. The formation of desmosine linkage joining two elastin chains, through the interaction of two previously synthesised *intra*-chain linkages.

Lent and Franzblau (1967) have estimated the individual cross-links in elastin, and have shown that desmosine, isodesmosine, lysinonorleucine and allysine aldol together with four unaltered lysine residues and the aldehydic precursor – δ-aminoadipic acid semialdehyde – allysine – account for between 38 and 41 potential lysine residues. Smith *et al.* (1968) reported between 42 and 45 lysine residues in soluble elastin derived from copper deficient pigs, where no cross-linkages have been formed, and hence the recovery of cross-links and unchanged lysine residues accounts for between 84 and 91 % of the lysine originally present.

The biosynthesis of elastin cross-links. Details of the hypothetical biosynthetic pathway whereby desmosines could be produced from four lysine residues were confirmed by Partridge *et al.* (1964) and Miller *et al.* (1964). They provided direct evidence for the sequence of reactions by a study of the incorporation of radioactivity into desmosines from ^{14}C-lysine. Miller *et al.* (1964) also showed that the only changes which could be observed in the amino-acid composition of elastin during the production of desmosines was a reduction in the amount of lysine recovered on hydrolysis. The research which has further confirmed the nature of the oxidative deamination process which transforms the elastin-bound lysine residues into δ-amino adipic acid semialdehyde (Martin and Pinell, 1968) has already been referred to in the section of the synthesis of collagen cross-links, (p. 90) hence it need not be discussed further here. Suffice it to say that the pathways whereby the more complex cross-links present in elastin are synthesised, are susceptible to inhibition at a far greater number of points. It is therefore, not surprising that not only is copper deficiency capable of preventing the formation of cross-links in elastin, but the administration of lathyrogens has a similar effect. As mentioned earlier, lathyrogens may interfere both by combining with amino groups, thus preventing Schiff's base formation, and by complexing the copper prevent the oxidative deamination of lysine by inhibiting lysine deaminase. One of the difficulties which arose from an acceptance of the oxidative deamination of lysine residues as a primary step in the pathway of desmosine synthesis, was the necessity to explain how one out of every four lysine residues remained unoxidised. In the early stages of these studies when all the desmosines were believed to join four separate polypeptide chains, it was possible to invoke steric effects which could exclude one chain from the sphere of activity of the lysine oxidase. However, the more recent concept of the primary synthesis of *intra*-chain linkages make this hypothesis completely untenable. Sandberg (1975) quotes Gray (unpublished observations) as suggesting that the fourth lysine of every set of four is protected by the presence of a tyrosine residue lying next to it in the sequence Lys-Ala-Ala-Lys-Tyr which is frequently repeated in the cross-linking region of the elastin molecule. Where lysine residues are surrounded by alanine residues as in the sequence Lys-Ala-Ala-Ala-Lys-Ala-Ala-Ala-etc., oxidation proceeds unchecked.

Desmosine linkages and maturation. The disappearance of lysine and the appearance of the desmosines in hydrolysates of elastins of increasing maturity has been studied by a number of workers. Labella and Vivian (1967) reported amino acid analyses for elastin preparations from human aortas ranging in age from a 14-week foetus to a 51-year old adult, and Rasmussen *et al.* (1975) for human aortic elastin from subjects aged 3–62. Values for desmosine, isodesmosine, merodesmosine and lysinonorleucine are always recorded as "lysine equivalents" or numbers of quarter-desmosines, third merodesmosines or half lysinonorleucines, since these fractions represent the appropriate proportion of each quadri-, tri- or bi-dentate molecule which can be appropriately attributed to each polypeptide chain.

According to Labella and Vivian (1967), the desmosine content increases from 3.2 quarter-residues/1000 residues in the elastin from a 14-week old foetus to a mean value of 7.1 at birth, and does not rise thereafter. Iso-desmosine on the other hand does not rise above a mean value of 5.6 quarter-residues, throughout postnatal life, although it is originally present in marginally higher amounts than desmosine in elastin from the aorta of the 14-week old foetus. Rasmussen *et al.* (1975) report far lower levels for both desmosines, ranging from 1.8 to 1.1 and 1.2 to 0.8. These values are in agreement with those found for other elastins, both by the same workers and by Serafini-Fracassini *et al.* (1975). These inconsistencies have not been fully explained, but may be due to the fact that the methods employed for the purification of elastin by the various groups of workers are markedly different. Labella and Vivian employed hot alkali treatment to remove collagen and other contaminants, Rasmussen *et al.* (1975) employed cold guanidine, formic acid and cyanogen bromide. It has long been proved that the results of alkali treatment are dependent on time, temperature and the ratio of alkali to solid elastic tissue (Wood, 1954, Hall, 1964). Prolonged treatment, or treatment at high liquor ratios, may easily result in total dissolution, and even under less drastic conditions, it is highly probable that portions of the molecule may be removed by main chain hydrolysis. Since the regions around the desmosines are stabilised by these linkages, the regions of the molecule which are lost will be desmosine free, and this could result in an increase in the apparent desmosine content of the residue. Even relatively mild methods of purification (Sykes and Partridge, 1974) result in the loss of 25% of the length of the molecule when compared with the values reported by Rasmussen *et al.* (1975) and it is quite possible that the degree of degradation induced by hot alkali treatment is even greater.

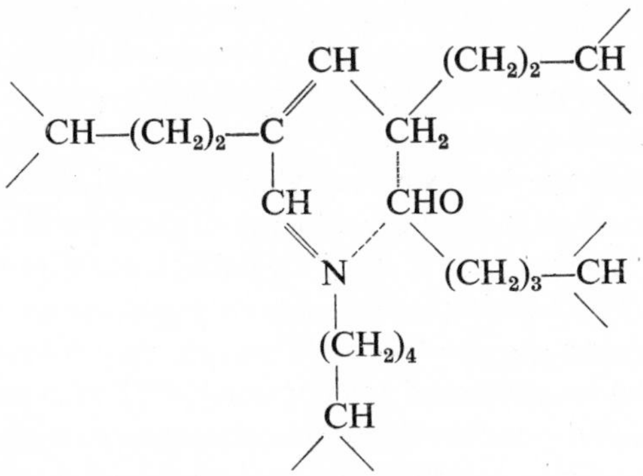

FIG. 56. The interaction of merodesmosine and allysine, to produce isodesmosine.

The preferential synthesis of the symmetrical cross-linkage – desmosine – rather than the asymmetrical one (Fig. 56) has been confirmed by a number of groups of workers (e.g. Ledvina and Bartos, 1968; Yu, 1970). This may indicate the greater ease with which cross-linkages are formed between merodesmosine and allysine when this entails the production of a carbon-nitrogen link than when the interaction which closes the pyridine ring is between two carbon atoms.

Another explanation for the preferential formation of one form of desmosine rather than the other has been suggested by Gray (Sandberg, 1975). He points out that if the concept of the primary synthesis of *intra*-chain allysine aldols and dehydrolysinonorleucines holds good and the final act of ring closure depends on the interaction of these two, then their individual structures can determine whether desmosine or isodesmosine is formed. Each of the bi-dentate molecules contains a single double bond, and can therefore, exist in either a *cis* or *trans* form. Oxidative condensation of the *cis* form of the aldol with the *trans* form of the aldimine will result in the formation of desmosine, whereas condensation of the opposite pair of isomers will permit the synthesis of isodesmosine. The production of the *cis* or *trans* forms of either *intra*-chain link will of course be dependent on the alignment of the two allysines in the one case, and the allysine and lysine in the other. If Gray's concept regarding the protection of one of the lysines from deamination due to the presence of an adjacent tyrosine, is correct, then the two ends of the aldimine *intra*-chain cross-links are invariably separated by two alanine residues whereas the two ends of the aldol are separated by three. These structural differences could determine whether *cis* or *trans* forms of the two structures were preferentially formed.

This whole hypothesis is very attractive but as yet there is no experimental evidence for it except for the identification of the appropriate *intra*-chain cross-linkages among the hydrolysis products of elastin.

Lysinonorleucine increases from 0.4 lysine equivalents/1000 residues during foetal growth to between 1 and 1.6 during the first 5 years of life (Labella and Vivian, 1967). Rasmussen *et al.* (1975) record lower levels for mature elastin, although the difference between the values reported by the two groups of workers are not as great as those which are apparent for the desmosines, probably indicating that lysinonorleucine linkages may be more widespread throughout the elastin molecules than are the more complex linkages. There may be evidence for a slight reduction in lysinonorleucine levels at ages above 5, but Yu (1971) does not record any appreciable fall even with severe atherosclerosis. Although this author does not record the age range of subjects with increasing degree of atherosclerosis, it may be assumed that those classified as having a severe grade of arterial involvement, will be among the more elderly.

Age changes in the other cross-linkages or cross-link intermediates, have not been recorded in detail, although Labella and Vivian report a steady decrease in two factors U_4 and U_5, which although unidentified, would appear to be allysine and allysine aldol. They are present in high concentration (9.6 residues/1000) in the 14 week foetus and fall rapidly during prenatal growth to 0.7 residues shortly after birth, but appear to continue to decrease in number but at a reduced rate, to reach a level of 0.2 residues/1000 at the age of 51.

The lysine content of foetal elastin falls rapidly during the last weeks before birth, and continues to fall slowly for the first year of life, but thereafter it would appear that all cross-linking which involves further oxidative deamination of this amino acid, has ceased.

Any further increase in the lysinonorleucine or merodesmosine content must occur at the expense of already preformed aldehydes, which are produced in quantities in excess of requirements during the period of rapid growth which precedes birth.

To return to the question of steric factors in cross-link formation, it must be borne in mind that the chances of a lysinonorleucine link being formed are far greater than are those of merodesmosine or desmosine synthesis assuming that these linkages join three or four chains, solely on account of the greater possibility of two rather than three or four chains becoming aligned in such a way that the necessary groups for aldol or Schiff's base formation are located within reacting distance of one another. Furthermore once any desmosine linkage is formed, four chains become more rigidly aligned and the chances of a second desmosine being synthesised are proportionally less. This probably explains why the linkages which involve fewer chains continue to be synthesised for over a longer period of time than the desmosines.

However, the recent analytical studies of Foster et al. (1973) and Gerber and Anwar (1974) which have demonstrated the existence of two-chain rather than four-chain linkages simplify the reaction pathway appreciably. Because of the relative location of the lysine residues to the adjacent lysine and tyrosine residues in the individual polypeptide chains, *intra*-chain aldol and aldimine linkages are formed at various points. The interaction of these pairs of linkages to form a desmosine-type structure, although involving the formation of two bonds only entails the juxtaposition of two chains, and hence is potentially as easily accomplished as in the formation of dehydrolysinonorleucine.

Until full quantitative assessments of the relative amounts of di-, tri- and tetra-chain linkages have been made, it will however, remain impossible to ascertain which of these hypotheses is correct.

Calcium cross-linkages. It has become increasingly apparent (Banga, 1966) that although the formation of lysine-derived cross-links falls off with age shortly after early youth, elastin continues to become progressively more resistant to enzymic attack over a much longer period of life. This anomaly has been ascribed to the introduction of another type of cross-link, evidence for which has arisen as the result of a study of the reaction between the enzyme elastase and its substrate, elastin (Hall, 1971).

Under normal circumstances in which an enzyme reacts with a soluble substrate, the former is usually larger in molecular weight and the reaction commences with the adsorption of the substrate onto reactive sites on the surface of the enzyme. In the degradation of elastin by elastase, the enzyme is of relatively low molecular weight (up to 25 000 daltons), whereas the substrate, being insoluble, is of infinite molecular weight. The normal kinetic relationships are therefore, not fully applicable and the approach and localisation of the enzyme on the surface of the substrate, rather than the reverse, is of major importance in the reaction (Hall, 1962).

It has been shown that both carboxyl and hydroxyl groups on both enzyme and substrate are essential for the formation of the enzyme/substrate complex (Hall and Czerkawski, 1962; Bagdy et al., 1960; Hall and El-Ridi, 1976a). The identity of the essential groups on both enzyme and substrate limits the number of possibilities for interaction and enzyme/substrate complex formation. Either pairs of ester linkages can be formed between enzyme and substrate or both may react with some common intermediate compound which, because of its bifunctional nature, can interact equally with reactive groups on both enzyme and substrate. Ester linkages are not common in the formation of enzyme/substrate complexes and esterification of the hydroxyl groups in the substrate effectively reduces the rate of elastolysis (Hall and Czerkawski, 1962). This would not in itself necessarily militate completely against the acceptance of this form of interaction were it not for positive identification of the existence of a possible intermediary substance through which the pairs of carboxyl and hydroxyl groups can be linked.

Chelating agents such as citrate (Hall, 1954), ethylene diamine tetraacetic acid (EDTA, Hall, 1954, 1969a, 1971) uramil diacetate, nitrolotriacetic acid, methylene diacetic acid and aminodiacetic acid (Graham, 1958) and certain metal EDTA complexes can inhibit elastolysis when administered directly to systems containing both enzyme and substrate. Conversely, calcium EDTA can activate the system (Cacciola et al., 1963; Hall, 1971). It has, therefore, been suggested that these various chelating agents act by stripping out from the enzyme/substrate system a metallic co-factor, which on the basis of the observations of Cacciola et al. (1963) and the subsequent studies by Hall (1971) is believed to be a co-ordinately bound calcium atom.

EDTA only inhibits elastolysis when it is present in the complete elastolysis system. No effect can be observed if either substrate or enzyme is separately pretreated with the reagent, which is then thoroughly removed by washing or dialysis before they are brought together. Either sufficient calcium is available from the glassware or the other reagents to re-activate the system, or EDTA is incapable of removing calcium present in either the substrate or the enzyme when it reacts on one or the other in the absence of the second half of the system. Yu and Blumenthal (1958) have in fact provided evidence that this latter possibility is the correct one by their demonstration that there are two forms of calcium bound to aortic elastic tissue, an EDTA-extractable fraction, and one which is resistant to extraction with the reagent.

Elastin does not lose calcium when treated with EDTA and when the whole elastolytic system is incubated in the presence of the chelating agent the latter is picked up from solution by the residual substrate, the amount which combines being proportional to the amounts of both enzyme and substrate in the reaction mixture.

On the basis of these observations it has been suggested (Hall, 1970a, 1973b) that both enzyme and substrate are in part cross-linked by co-ordinately bound calcium atoms. The calcium atom is capable of building up a co-ordination sphere with its own electrons and others which it either gathers from carboxyl groups or shares with hydroxyl groups (Fig. 57). The fact that this co-ordination complex is stable even in the presence of EDTA implies that the co-ordination constants of both enzyme and substrate have values which are higher than that which is characteristic of the calcium-EDTA complex.

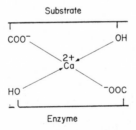

FIG. 57. The role of the co-ordinated calcium atoms in the production of the enzyme/substrate complex in elastolysis.

The amounts of EDTA taken up by the residual elastin when added to a system containing both enzyme and substrate is not only proportional to the relative concentrations of these two separate components of the system, but also to the calcium content of each. Elastin preparations containing between 0.012 and 0.060% calcium pick up between 0.6 and 1.4 μmoles of EDTA from a solution containing 2 μmoles of this reagent when incubated in the presence of an elastase preparation containing 0.032% calcium (Hall, 1971). Similarly, between 0.48 and 1.69 μmoles of EDTA combine with elastin containing 0.012% calcium when incubated with elastase containing between 0.02 and 0.141% calcium.

It has been suggested, therefore, that some of the carboxyl and hydroxyl groups in elastin are cross-linked by calcium, leaving some of the groupings free. When this cross-linked substrate is allowed to react with elastase which is free of calcium, the co-ordination shell is disrupted and reformed with electrons derived from the carboxyl and hydroxyl groups of the enzyme.

$$\text{Substrate–Ca–Substrate} + \text{Elastase} \rightarrow \text{Substrate–Ca–Elastase} \qquad (1)$$

$$(\text{S–Ca–S} + \text{E} \rightarrow \text{S–Ca–E} + \text{S})$$

Similarly cross-linked elastase can react with those parts of the substrate which contain free carboxyl and hydroxyl groups with a concomitant inter-change of electrons – this time between enzyme and substrate.

$$\text{E–Ca–E} + \text{S} \rightarrow \text{E–Ca–S} + \text{E} \qquad (2)$$

The enzyme/substrate complexes formed by the two types of reaction defined by equations 1 and 2 are essentially identical (but see p. 99) although they will of necessity be formed by the interaction of different sets of reactive groupings on both substrate and enzyme. If a bifunctional chelating agent such as EDTA is allowed to react with the elastin/elastase system at the moment when the substrate cross-link is on the point of being cleaved by the monomeric form of the enzyme or when the dimeric form of the enzyme is being cleaved by free carboxyl and hydroxyl groups on the substrate, it will be able to insert itself between two "nascent" enzymes or two "nascent" substrate molecules containing calcium atoms which are surrounded by incomplete co-ordination shells.

$$2(\text{E–Ca–E}) + \text{V} \xrightarrow{\ 2\text{S}\ } \text{E–Ca–V–Ca–E} + 2\text{E} \qquad (3)$$

$$2(\text{S–Ca–S}) + \text{V} \xrightarrow{\ 2\text{E}\ } \text{S–Ca–V–Ca–S} + 2\text{S} \qquad (4)$$

$$\text{V} = \text{chelating agent, EDTA or Versene}$$

The involvement of substrate in the first of these equations (3) or enzyme in the second (4) is merely that of a catalyst since this component does not become involved in the final complex. The incorporation of the chelating agent in the dimeric form of the enzyme or in the substrate molecule, irreversibly removes one or other of these components of the reaction mixture from the system. This is of course only true where it is possible to separate cross-linked and non-cross-linked species from one another completely. The enzyme can be fractionated into two such species (see below) but while cross-linkages may be incorporated into one area of the substrate, which will therefore react as S-Ca-S, other regions may still contain free carboxyl and hydroxyl groups, and hence effectively take part in the reaction as S. Under these conditions interaction of such a mixed substrate with the dimeric enzyme can follow a more complicated pathway (equations 5, 6 and 7) involving the release of "nascent" molecules of calcium bound enzyme and substrate, the latter being released from the fully co-ordinated region of the substrate molecule by molecules of the monomeric form of the enzyme which in turn is released from the dimeric form by non-cross-linked regions of the substrate. These two nascent molecules may then interact with the ethylene diamine tetraacetic acid to give an enzyme substrate complex in which the two components are separated by an EDTA residue.

$$E-Ca-E \xrightarrow{\;S\;} E-Ca'+E \tag{5}$$

$$S-Ca-S \xrightarrow{\;E\;} S-Ca'+S \tag{6}$$

$$E-Ca+S+Ca'+V \rightarrow E-Ca-V-Ca-S \tag{7}$$

Hall (1971) and Cacciola et al. (1963) have shown that that amount of ethylene diamine tetraacetic acid added to an elastolysis system can determine the type of response. Low concentrations result in the activation of the system, and this is followed by inhibition as the concentration is increased. Activation may be due to the fact that the insertion of an EDTA residue between enzyme and substrate will permit the removal of certain elements of steric hindrance which may normally occur when the enzyme protein is located directly on the surface of the substrate.

From the differences which can be observed in the uptake of EDTA which depends on the calcium levels of both enzyme and substrate, it can be deduced that the calcium content of the two components of the system will also determine the rate of elastolysis. Elastin preparations can be modified by treatment with solutions of calcium ethylene diamine tetraacetate to produce modified substrates with varying rates of susceptibility to elastase. An elastin preparation from ox aorta initially containing 0.012% calcium when treated with Ca-EDTA at concentrations of from 1 to 28 μmolar increased its sensivity to an elastase preparation containing 0.032% calcium at all Ca-EDTA concentrations up to 4 μmolar. Thereafter the rate of elastolysis fell by 2% for every 1 micromolar increment in Ca-EDTA concentration. Although these observations themselves might prove of considerable use in determining the changes in co-ordinately bound calcium content of elastin with increasing age, even better evidence can be obtained by a study of the relative elastolytic effects of elastase preparations purified according to their calcium content.

Sialic acid containing linkages. In addition to elastin and collagen and other proteins, aortic tissue contains about 2% of carbohydrate (Hall et al., 1952) whereas skin contains 0.05% (Fleischmajer et al., 1973) and the nuchal ligaments of cattle 0.5% (Hall et al., 1952). An appreciable proportion of these carbohydrate molecules can be separated from elastin during the normal purification procedures, but an undefined carbohydrate element is retained along with the elastin even after most methods of treatment (Loeven, 1960). Czerkawski (1962) isolated a fragment containing the elastin-sugar linkage, using very mild conditions, and reported that a major component of this material was the amino sugar, sialic acid.

Treatment of bovine aortic tissue with pepsin, trypsin and collagenase removed virtually all the collagen, non-collagenous protein and glycosaminoglycan leaving a residue which amounted to 50% of the total dry weight of the aortic tissue. Over 90% of this material could be dissolved by elastase (the calcium-poor insoluble species, cf. p. 99), to give high and low molecular weight fractions. The high molecular weight material contained 0.5% of a substance giving the usual reactions for sugar, but contained no glucosamine or galactosamine, merely sialic and hexuronic acids. The sialic acid could be determined by the thiobarbiturate method of Aminoff (1961) after partial hydrolysis with 0.1N sulphuric acid for 1 h at 80° C. This liberation of the active group of the sialic acid by hydrolysis did not completely remove the polysaccharide from the protein, since the sugar residues could not be separated by dialysis. No sialic acid could be detected by the thiobarbiturate method after dialysis, although its reactivity with this reagent could be restored after a second period of treatment with acid. Czerkawski concluded that contrary to its normal terminal position in carbohydrate chains, sialic acid was in this instance bound to the elastin protein by two linkages, thus functioning essentially as a potential cross-linking agent. Although present in relatively low concentration (about 1 mole/10^5 g elastin), sialic acid may be assumed to be an important constituent of the elastin molecule, since its presence prevents further degradation by elastase.

Hall (1967) has shown that the sialic acid content of bovine aortic elastin purified by hot decinormal alkali rises from 0.08% in foetal tissue, to 0.26% in a 4-year old animal. Thereafter the sialic acid content falls dramatically to a level of only 0.04% in 7-year old animals. This potential cross-linking agent therefore differs from the structural glycoproteins (see below) which are present in highest concentration in the foetus, and fall steadily thereafter.

Other cross-links in connective tissue components

Bifunctional aldehydes. Milch (1963) studied the effect of various bifunctional aldehydes on the physical and biochemical properties of collagen, and observed a basic similarity between the properties of the modified protein, and that present in ageing tissue. On the basis of this he suggested that certain intermediary metabolites of carbohydrate metabolism which were ubiquitous in the body could be responsible for the cross-linkages which altered the properties of ageing collagen. Of those aldehydes which he studied, dl-glyceraldehyde, formaldehyde and glyoxal produced the greatest effect. Bjorksten (1968) points out that cross-linking agents can be of two types, slow reacting and instantaneous, and the bi-functioal aldehyde residues normally present in the body could be of either category. However, no further evidence has been produced since Milch's original observations to confirm that cross-linkages of this type are present in the normal aged tissues of the body, but it might prove difficult to liberate easily metabolisable groupings of this type by hydrolysis of heavily cross-linked protein, without destroying the linking molecule itself.

Dityrosine and quinones. A biphenolic compound formed by the interaction of two tyrosine molecules has been identified in acid hydrolysates of resilin, the rubber-like protein in the wing ligaments of insects (Anderson, 1964, 1966). Labella *et al.* (1967) studying the incorporation of ^{14}C-tyrosine into the elastin of the aortas of chick embryos, detected radioactivity not only in the tyrosine region of the amino acid chromatogram, but also in two other peaks, one of which they were subsequently able to identify as being due to a compound, the properties of which were identical with those of the di-tyrosine isolated by Anderson. The di-tyrosine is intensly fluorescent, and may account in part at least for the native fluorescence of the elastin molecule. Keeley *et al.* (1969) have isolated di-tyrosine from an alkali soluble extract of chick aorta and bovine ligamentum nuchae, and have shown it to be present at a concentration of about 10 residues per 100 000 total residues in this protein. In elastin itself it is present in smaller amounts (3 residues/100 000). Labella (1971) has suggested that the presence of this small amount of di-tyrosine may be due to the contamination of the whole elastin protein with the glycoprotein microfibrils (Ross and Bornstein, 1969, cf. p. 112) which are present in larger proportion in the immature elastic fibre than in mature elastin. Labella *et al.* (1968) were also able to identify di-tyrosine in preparations of soluble collagen from rat-skin. Tyrosine only occurs in the telopeptide regions of collagen, and an interaction between residues in the telopeptide regions of adjacent tropocollagen molecules could bind them together by the formation of *inter*-chain linkages (Dabbous, 1966). The addition of peroxidase and peroxide, to solutions of soluble collagen results in the rapid formation of a clear protein gel (Labella *et al.*, 1968) which appeared to be formed by the production of one di-tyrosine linkage for approximately every five collagen molecules. Removal of the telopeptide by trypsin treatment prevented gel formation. Fujimori (1966) was also able to induce cross-link formation in soluble collagen by irradiation with ultra-violet light. Highly fluorescent photoproducts were formed, and it would appear likely that among these was included di-tyrosine.

Another form of oxidative modification of the tyrosine residue can result in the formation of quinones. The quinone tanning of protein-chitin complexes has been shown to occur in the cuticle of insects (Brunet and Kent, 1955), the quinones either arising from the oxidation of tyrosine residues in the protein, or from the circulation. In the human, the elastase resistant portion of the elastic fibre and the insoluble mature form of collagen become increasingly fluorescent with increasing age. In both collagen and elastin, this fluorescent material shows spectra which are similar to those of quinone (Labella *et al.*, 1967; Labella, 1962) and this material increases with age inversely as the tyrosine content falls.

It would appear most likely that the continuing formation of cross-links in mature collagen, already cross-linked by the lysine derived linkages reviewed earlier, results from the production of quinones which are formed from phenolic residues already present in the collagen. However, the intervention of circulating quinones such as have been postulated in the hardening of insect cuticle cannot be ruled out. Several polyhydric alcohols, both aromatic and aliphatic have been shown to increase the aggregation of soluble collagen. For these polyalcohols to be effective, an oxidative step is required and notable in the list provided by Grant and Alburn (1965) and Labella (1971) are the ubiquitous catecholamines and the abnormal metabolic product of phenylalanine and tyrosine, homogentisic acid, which binds strongly to collagenous structures in subjects suffering from alkaptonuria.

Metallic cross-links. The normal animal body is capable of dealing satisfactorally with iron, zinc, magnesium, manganese, copper and calcium. Under certain circumstances, however, even some of these metals may accumulate in tissues, when their polyvalence enable them to link two or more protein chains together. Calcium, for instance, has been shown to combine with elastin with the production of co-ordination shells of electrons derived partly from the metal, and partly from carboxyl and hydroxyl groups in adjacent elastin chains (p. 130). Others may accumulate if the normal mechanisms for their homeostasis are inoperative. Thus copper accumulates in Wilson's disease and may in part at least appear as cross-linkages in connective tissues, similarly iron deposits in the tissues as haemosiderin and part at least of this may be bound to the tissue components.

Glycoproteins and proteoglycans

General considerations

The polysaccharide complexes of connective tissue can be divided into two distinct groups, glycoproteins consisting of protein molecules to which monosaccharides or oligosaccharides are bound by covalent linkages, and on the other hand, proteoglycans consisting of polysaccharide protein complexes in which the polysaccharide constitutes a major part of the whole. In the main, the polysaccharide components of the proteoglycans consist of polymers of disaccharide units containing one or other of the various types of amino sugar coupled to either a neutral sugar residue or a uronic acid residue. These polysaccharides, termed glycosamino-glycans (GAG) (Jeanloz, 1960), may derive their negative charge from the uronic acid residue, or may be sulphated.

Hyaluronic acid. The main un-sulphated GAG is hyaluronic acid, which consists of a chain of sugar residues made up of alternate molecules of D-glucuronic acid and 2-acetamide-2-deoxy-D-glucose (N-acetyl-glucosamine) linked alternately 1–4 and 1–3. Hyaluronic acid is one of the main polysaccharide constituents of connective tissue ground substance, being

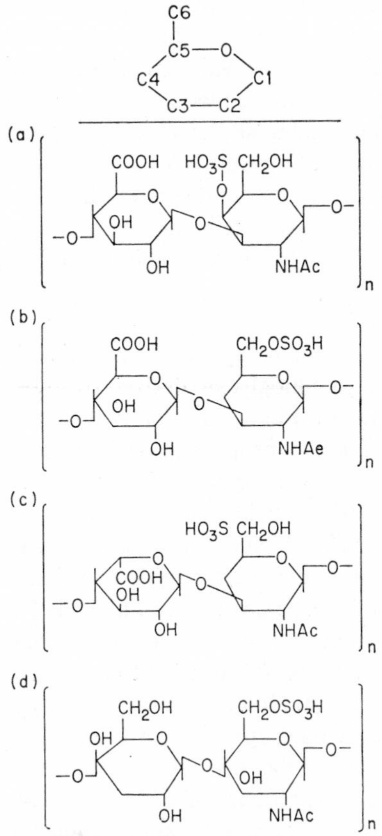

FIG. 58. Structures of various sulphated glycosaminoglycans. (a) chondroitin sulphate-4; (b) chondroitin sulphate-6; (c) dermatan sulphate; (d) keratan sulphate.

present at concentrations of between 0.03% in human skin to 0.36% in human synovial fluid, but may be present at levels of up to 0.75% in certain specific tumours and in the adult rooster comb.

There is considerable controversy as to whether hyaluronic acid exists in the form of a proteoglycan. Most proteins can be removed from HA by mild physical methods, but Sandson and Hamerman (1962) separated a fraction from synovial fluid by electrophoresis and adsorption chromatography which contained 2% protein, and Laurent (1970) obtained a protein-containing fraction from rooster comb. The hyaluronic acid macromolecule, whether in association with protein or not, has been implicated in the lubrication of joints in view of its relatively high concentration in synovial fluid. Rodin *et al.* (1970), however, fractionated bovine synovial fluid by density gradient sedimentation equilibration (Silpananta *et al.*, 1968). They were able to separate the fluid into three fractions, only the middle one, which banded at a density of 1.63 g cm^{-3}, contained hyaluronic acid. It was, however, the less dense third fraction which provided lubricating activity similar to that of intact synovial fluid, reducing the coefficient of friction between two surfaces of bovine metatarsal-phalangeal joint cartilage to 50% of that observed with buffer alone. Since no HA could be identified in this fraction, it was assumed by these workers that this GAG was without anti-frictional effect in the joint and hence any reduction in concentration with increasing age could not be responsible for increasing joint stiffness.

Sulphated glycosaminoglycans

All vertebrate cartilage, and many other connective tissues contain the same types of sulphated glycosaminoglycan, derived from the basic repeating units of chondroitin sulphate (CS) and dermatan sulphate (DS) keratan sulphate (KS) (Fig. 58). The relative proportions of these three types and their degree of sulphation vary with species site and age. The two chondroitin sulphates CS–4 and CS–6 have an identical repeating polysaccharide backbone, but differ in the positions at which they are sulphated. The repeating disaccharide unit consists of a molecule of glucuronic acid linked 1–3 to a molecule of galactosamine. Pairs of these residues are linked 1–4 to make up the entire chain. It was originally felt that each of these polysaccharides could exist as a separate entity, and was probably attached to its own specific protein to provide a separate proteoglycan. However, more recently it has been shown that a considerable degree of heterogeneity exists in proteoglycans as they are separated from tissue and it has been shown that not only can this heterogeneity extend to differing amounts of CS-4 and CS-6 in one proteoglycan molecule, but also to the presence of keratan sulphate as well.

Individual chondroitin disaccharides may exist in an unsulphated state, or may be substituted at the C-4 carbon atom of the galactosamine residue to give a CS-4 molecule or at the C-6 carbon atom of the galactosamine residue to give CS-6. Sometimes both carbon atoms may be sulphated, and sections of chondroitin in any one proteoglycan molecule may be hypersubstituted, containing sulphate residues in addition at either C-2 or C-3 of the glucuronic acid residue.

Keratan disaccharides may also lack sulphate entirely, or may carry sulphate residues at the C-6 carbon of either the glucosamine or the galactose residues.

Dermatan sulphate first isolated by Meyer and Chaffee (1941), was shown by Hoffman et al. (1956) and Cifonelli et al. (1958) to consist of a co-polymer of iduronic acid and galactosamine. However, about 5–10% of the uronic acid residues have been shown to consist of the epimer glucuronic acid (Cifonelli et al., 1958) and the hybrid nature of the glycosaminoglycan itself, as opposed to the hybidisation of the proteoglycan molecule referred to above, has been confirmed by the isolation of a tetrasaccharide from a hyaluronidase digest of dermatan sulphate (Fransson and Roden, 1967) which contained both uronic acid species.

The sulphation of the dermatan molecule takes place invariably on the acetylgalactosamine residue, in either positions 4 or 6. In the skin the hexoamines are substituted in C-4 whether they are adjacent to the iduronic or the glucuronic acid residues. In the umbilical cord, however, both C-4 and C-6 substituted hexosamines exist along the length of the molecule (Fransson, 1970) depending on the distribution of uronic acid species.

Dermatan sulphate because of its presence together with chondroitin sulphates in the skin, was originally classified as chrondroitin sulphate B, and in early papers the term chondroitin sulphate A is used to refer to CS-6 and chondroitin sulphate C to CS-4.

The problem of the macromolecular structure of the proteoglycans has been studied by various groups of workers; among whom Buddecke et al. (1967); Mathews (1962) and Tsiganos and Muir (1973) have approached the subject from a variety of points of view. The proteochondroitin sulphate of bovine nasal cartilage, in which 94% of the polysaccharide consists of one or other form of CS, has a weight average molecular weight of c. 2.78×10^6 daltons and a number average molecular weight of c. 0.55×10^6 daltons, indicating a considerable degree of molecular polydispersity. Buddecke et al. (1973b) have combined the results of studies by Hascall and Sajdera (1969) and Rosenberg et al. (1970) with observations of their own to explain this polydispersity. In the electron microscope it can be seen that at least two forms of proteoglycan macromolecule exist. A central polypeptide chain, which may be either 1790–1900 Å or 3200–3400 Å in length, is substituted at regular intervals along its length by either 20–22 or 34 polysaccharide side chains, each 530 Å in length. These polysaccharide chains are about 42 disaccharide units in length, and although each one may represent either a CS or KS structure, depending on the nature of the tissue from which the proteoglycan is derived, the same protein core may carry a mixture of glycosaminoglycans.

Tsiganos and Muir (1973) have reported that proteoglycans may be aggregated with one another by means of a glycoprotein link. The bonds linking this glycoprotein to the individual proteoglycans can be cleaved with 4M guanidine and separated from them by density gradient equilibration (Hascall and Sadjera, 1969). They were able to observe a quite marked alteration in the degree of aggregation of the proteoglycans of the laryngeal cartilage of pigs between the ages of 9 months and 5 years. Proteoglycans, by virtue of their charge, may react directly with collagen structures (Mathews, 1970) to form macromolecular complexes of modified function. Since age changes occur in the glycosaminoglycan content of polysaccharide-rich tissues (p. 43) the combination of different types of GAG to the collagen may alter the physical properties of the protein in different ways. Mathews (1973) has suggested for instance that the substitution of proteoglycan typical of the costal cartilage of a 50-year old subject for that characteristic of a 2-year old might be expected to lower the values of such parameters as the electrostatic interaction of the complex, its osmotic pressure, cation binding capacity and Donnan effect, whilst permitting greater penetration and diffusion of solutes. These are in fact the types of alteration which can be observed in the properties of cartilage with increasing age.

Glycoproteins

Chapman (1966) has suggested that there may be an upper limit to the size of molecular aggregate which can be derived from tropocollagen molecules alone. Structures of greater diameter may require the involvement of proteoglycans and glycoproteins. Steven (1964) and Steven and Jackson (1967) have shown that when these polysaccharides are removed from collagenous tissues, the macromolecular collagen molecules disperse due to cleavage of the cohesive forces holding them together. Heikkinen (1973) has published a schematic representation of the structure of collagen fibres in which he suggests that some of the linkages between tropocollagen polymers may be via proteoglycans, as suggested above, whereas other groups of protein polymers may be linked via glycoproteins.

Anderson and Jackson (1972) have isolated two glycoprotein fractions from tendon, one by extraction with sodium chloride solution, the other with 3M magnesium chloride. Separation from collagen and proteoglycans could then be accomplished by density gradient centrifugation. The protein moieties were rich in glutamic and aspartic acids and contained little hydroxyproline or hydroxylysine, although glycoprotein B which required the higher ionic strength for its extraction must have contained at least part of the collagen molecule to which it was attached since its hydroxyproline content was 24 residues/1000.

Neither fraction is homogenous, and the presence of a selection of hexoses and pentoses may not imply that all of these are combined in the same molecule.

Age changes in the glycosaminoglycan and glycoprotein content of various tissues

Cartilage. Matthews and his colleagues have studied the glycosaminoglycan composition of the cartilages of a variety of species and tissues, and the changes which occur in the repeating periods of the individual CS and KS types which make up the whole of the cartilage polysaccharide. Matthews and Hinds (1963) for instance have studied the composition of the glycosaminoglycans in the cranial cartilage of the frog and have shown that the un-sulphated periods which represent 40% of the total in young tadpoles decrease to 10% in the late tadpole stage and are completely lacking in the adult frog. On the other hand CS-4 periods build up from 40% of the total to 70% during growth and metamorphosis, whereas CS-6 periods which increase during larval growth, tend to fall after metamorphosis.

Differences in the way the glycosaminoglycans vary from tissue to tissue within one species can also be observed by comparison of studies by Shulman and Meyer (1968) on vertebral cartilage and by Matthews (1965, 1967) on epiphyseal cartilage, both in the chick. The epiphyseal cartilage in the 14 day embryonic chick consists in the main of CS-6 and unsulphated periods. At a later stage before hatching, both these species of glycosaminoglycan tend to be replaced by CS-4 species, and in the growing hatched chick, the unsulphated periods disappear completely to be replaced after 17 weeks by small amounts of keratan sulphate.

The composition of the costal cartilage of the rat changes slightly with age, CS-4 increasing and CS-6 decreasing over the first 9 months of life. Thereafter there are only minor changes although the glycan content of the cartilage as a whole falls dramatically (Weil *et al.*, 1969). As will be seen below this development is unusual, in that there is no synthesis of keratan sulphate with ageing such as occurs in other animals. This failure to observe KS periods in the proteoglycans from rat tissue may merely be indicative of the fact that the 14 month period of growth studied by Mathews and Glagov (1966) is not sufficient to render the animals truly old.

The composition of the proteoglycan prepared from human costal cartilage (Mathews and Glagov, 1966) changes quite dramatically with age (Fig. 59). During foetal growth CS-4 and CS-6 together make up between 80 and 100% of the total glycan, sharing this total equally between them. The remaining 20% in a mid-term foetus consists of non-sulphated chondroitin periods, but the component is progressively sulphated during the remaining months of foetal growth, and has completely disappeared by birth. After birth the CS-6 component falls very slightly throughout life, from 50 to 38% in the ensuing 70 years. The CS-4 fraction, however, after the first 2 or 3 years of postnatal life drops rapidly to reach about 5% by 40 years of age. It does not fall further, remaining at this small but finite level for the remainder of the life span. These reductions in CS species are offset by a rapid rise in keratan sulphate over the period 3 or 4 to 40 years of age. At birth this constituent is completely lacking, by 40 years of age it represents some 60% of the total glycan.

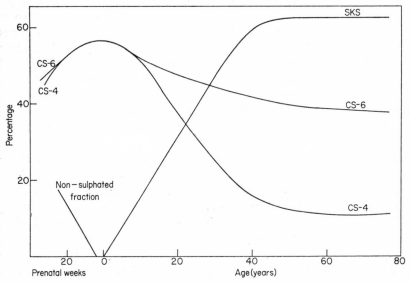

FIG. 59. Age changes in the proportions of different sulphated glycosaminoglycan units in the proteoglycans from human costal cartilage (after Mathews, 1973).

The two forms of CS in human knee joint cartilage (Greiling and Bauman, 1973) do not have the same time dependence as in costal cartilage. The CS-4 type falls linearly by 2 μg/g cartilage/year between birth and 85 years of age. The CS-6 type however, increases at 0.5 μg/g/year up to the age of 70 and then falls away at almost the same rate as the CS-4. If these findings are converted to percentage composition of the total glycan content so as to be comparable with the observations of Mathews represented in Fig. 59, it can be seen that the two lines rise and fall respectively at increasing rates above 40 years of age (Fig. 60).

Changes in CS content and in the CS/KS ratio may be indicative of true ageing phenomena. Such changes can in fact be accelerated by the intravenous administration of papain to rabbits (Halpern *et al.*, 1965) when proteoglycan staining like keratan sulphate surrounds the cells in the cartilage of the rabbit ear. Since papain produces an accelerated catabolism of the cartilage constituents, the experimental procedure is in fact merely speeding up the normal remodelling processes of the body. After repeated depletion of the tissue proteins, "ageing" phenomena similar to those reported by Leutert and Kreutz (1964) in normally ageing cartilage can be observed. These workers observed different rates for the appearance of such changes in different types of cartilage, tracheal cartilage being the slowest to change, and thyroideal cartilage the most rapid. The types of change observed by Leutert (1964) are vascularisation, fibrosis and calcification.

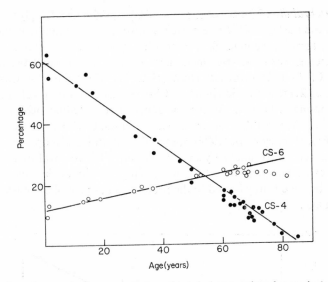

FIG. 60. Age changes in the percentages of total glycosaminoglycans in human knee cartilage represented by the C-4 and C-6 forms of chondroitin sulphate. (Calculated from the figures of Greiling and Bauman, 1973.)

Dermis. The amount of glycosaminoglycan present in dermis falls dramatically with age (Fleischmajer *et al.*, 1972) from 722 µg uronic acid/g dry weight of dermis to 226 µg/g between birth and old age (a group of six people aged between 67 and 96 years). Hexosamines are present at 5.8 times the concentration of uronic acid in the new-born, and at 10.2 times this concentration in the old age group. This may represent a change in the ratios of the individual glycosaminoglycans over and above the differences in hyaluronic acid and dermatan sulphate levels which have been reported by Fleischmajer *et al.* (1972). The hyaluronic acid remains relatively unbound to protein throughout life, being easily extractable in 1M sodium chloride. Dermatan sulphate on the other hand, becomes more firmly bound throughout postnatal life, the percentage of inextractable fraction increasing from 49 to 71 % between 5 and 96 years. At birth, however, the majority of the dermatan sulphate, which is present in high concentration in such tissue is in the bound form.

This could indicate that the synthesis of dermatan sulphate is reduced with increasing age, leaving that portion which has been firmly bound to the tissue intact. Pearson (1970), however, has suggested that the total dermatan sulphate content of the various layers of dermis remains essentially constant, and that the alterations in fibre thickness which are dependent on increased dermatan sulphate: hyaluronic acid levels are in fact occasioned by a reduction in hyaluronic acid level.

Intervertebral disc. The concentration of CS-4, CS-6 and KS glycosamino-glycans in the nucleus of the intervertebral disc, which is initially higher than that in the annulus, changes its composition with age. The total content of GAG decreases with age (Buddecke and Seigoleits, 1964) and the ratio of CS-4 and CS-6 to KS decreases from 1:1 to 1:4 whilst the CS-4/CS-6 ratio changes from 2:1 to a situation in which CS-6 represents the major chondroitin-based component. Over a shorter age range, but including two values for foetal discs, Szirmai (1970) records a change in the CS/KS ratio from 5:2 to 6:7 (Fig. 61). Happey *et al.* (1974) observed a fall in the glycoproteins of the nucleus between birth and 70 years of age, after the removal of the glyco-saminoglycans. This may reflect the increasing inability of the glycosamino-glycans to become firmly bound to the protein component of the nucleus with increasing age.

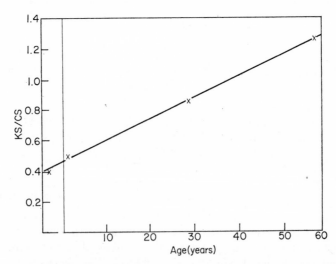

FIG. 61. The ratio of keratin sulphate to chrondroitin sulphate glycans in human intervertebral discs from an 18-week foetus to a 58-year old adult.

5

The Metabolism of Connective Tissue

Synthesis

Age changes in the activity of fibroblasts

The human diploid fibroblast has been studied fully by a number of workers during the past few years. Hayflick (1970) showed that cultured fibroblasts from young donors could produce up to fifty generations of daughter cells, whereas similar cultures of cells from more elderly subjects could not be sub-cultured for more than half this number of doublings. Holliday and Tarrant (1972) and Lewis and Tarrant (1972) have demonstrated that the failure of old cells to maintain the full number of generations typical of cells from young adults is due to the accumulation of error proteins in accordance with the theory originally propounded by Orgel (1963). Altered proteins have been detected among the tissue components synthesised by fibroblasts from ageing lung tissue (Holliday and Tarrant, 1972) but Nemetschek had suggested earlier that "old" protein is produced by fibroblasts from old individuals and that newly formed collagen from an old animal has a faster ageing rate than that from a young animal, thus implying that the altered metabolism of collagen in old age is dependent on the accumulation of errors in the fibroblasts themselves. There is, however, in addition an appreciable amount of evidence which is in favour of a programmed pathway for the ageing of connective tissue.

Collagen has recently been shown to exist in different forms, not only in various tissues, but also in the same tissue at different periods throughout life. Thus for instance, whereas adult skin collagen consists of the $(\alpha 1)_2 \alpha 2$ type, human skin from a new-born child also contains the $(\alpha 1)_3$ type. If one assumes that a separate gene is responsible for the development of the messenger RNA required for the synthesis of each of these types of α-chain, the change from the dual type of collagen in the infant skin to the single type present in the adult, must involve the turning off of the particular gene which is responsible for the synthesis of the $(\alpha 1)_3$ type. Another explanation could be that the two types of collagen are each synthesised by a separate strain of fibroblast, but such a concept merely pushes the control reaction one stage further back. It is still necessary to postulate a control mechanism to activate one strain of cell at the expense of the other.

145

Related changes occur in granuloma tissue which has been induced in animals of various ages (Heikkinen *et al.*, 1971; Schmitt and Beneke, 1971). All those factors which determine the particular metabolic activities of the fibroblasts which are responsible for the growth of the granuloma, such as oxygen consumption, the activity of the enzymes of the citric acid cycle and other enzymes involved in glycolysis and the pentosephosphate cycle, together with those involved in the *in vitro* synthesis of collagen by slices of the newly synthesised tissue, are depressed in old age. In young animals peak activity occurs around 20 days following the implantation of the granulomagenic agent (Fig. 62). In old animals the peak which is lower and broader does not develop until nearly 10 days later. The repression of enzymic activity which occurs in young tissue 30+ days following implantation is most probably due to an alteration in the site on the DNA molecule to which its accompanying histone is bound. The relatively slow reduction in activity of elderly granuloma tissue during the later periods of its growth may well be due to the existence of co-valent linkages between DNA and histone which are not easily broken. This will prevent the redistribution of histone along the length of the chromatin strand which is necessary for the repression of one gene locus and the de-repression of another. Hahn (1964) has suggested that the relative inextract-ability of DNA from elderly tissues is due to the development of more resis-tant linkages of this type between DNA and histone and Heikkinen *et al.*

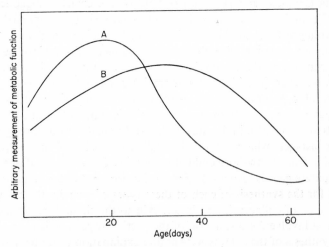

FIG. 62. Changes in the "metabolic function" of granulomas during sixty days fol-lowing the implantation of the initiating substance into young (A) and old (B) animals. The term "metabolic function" covers such factors as the synthesis of collagen and non-collagenous proteins, oxygen consumption and the activity of glycolytic enzymes (after Heikkinen, 1973).

(1971) have demonstrated a marked reduction in the ease with which DNA can be extracted from granuloma tissue which has been induced in elderly rats.

Changes in the growth of collagen fibres

Characteristic changes occur in the rate at which collagen fibres are synthesised in the body, depending on alterations in the activity of those enzyme systems which are involved in the reaction. Heikkinen (1969) has shown that enzyme systems in the cells of rat tail tendon decrease linearly with the log of the age of the animal over the period from 2.5 to 100 weeks. One enzyme, protocollagen proline hydroxylase, which is responsible for the introduction of the hydroxyl group into proline residues which have already been incorporated into the protocollagen molecule, falls to one tenth the value apparent in foetal tissue during the first 100 days of life. This age change, is accompanied by a reduction in the overall rate of collagen synthesis as measured by the rate at which radioactive proline is incorporated into 0.45M NaCl-soluble collagen fraction. These findings indicate that collagen synthesis both at the *proto*- and *tropo*-collagen stages of development decrease with increasing age. Similar changes are apparent in human skin collagen over an even longer portion of the total life span (Bakerman, 1962; Uitto, 1971). The activity of protocollagen proline hydroxylase expressed in terms of dpm/mg of ^{14}C-hydroxyproline formed during incubation, falls from 14 to 2 between 1 and 50 years of age, and this is reflected by an 85% decrease in soluble collagen formation.

The other hydroxylase of importance in collagen synthesis – lysine hydroxylase – also decreases with ageing (Kivirikko *et al.*, 1972; Heikkinen, 1973) thus limiting the number of hydroxylysine residues available for the specific cross-links which form on these groupings.

The liberation of the tropocollagen molecule from the registration peptides which locate the procollagen molecules during the synthesis of the triple helix is also age dependent (Lapierre *et al.*, 1973). The activity of the enzyme which splits the terminal peptides from each pro-α-chain – procollagen peptidase – decreases with age.

Glycosaminoglycan synthesis

The assembly of macromolecular glycosaminoglycans from the constituent sugars, and the combination of the GAG molecules with the protein core, to give one or other form of proteoglycan (p. 137), depends on the oxidation, amination and transfer of individual sugar residues to the growing molecular chain. Dorfman (1970) has proposed a scheme for the synthesis of the glycosaminoglycan in which at least seven transferase enzymes and the appropriate number of oxidases and deaminases required to synthesise each sugar residue from glucose, are involved.

Rodén (1970) reviewing the possible mechanisms for this complex synthetic process, showed that the first stage consisted of the transfer of a xylose residue to a suitable serine hydroxyl group on the protein core. The xylose is brought to the site of synthesis in the cell in the form of its uridine nucleotide, the synthesis of which together with that of other UDP-sugars is now well understood (Kornfeld *et al.*, 1964). The fact that the initiation step involves the transfer of a xylose residue to the protein core indicates that the proteoglycan as a whole is the fundamental entity rather than the separate glycosaminoglycan molecule which then combines with the core protein. Subsequent sugar molecules for transfer to the growing glycosaminoglycan chain are synthesised from UDP-glucose. In view of the number of enzyme systems which are required for the complete synthesis of, for example, a hybrid CS-4/CS-6 proteoglycan it is not surprising that age changes occur in the rates of proteoglycan synthesis. Evidence has been reported which indicates that a number of the enzymes of these pathways are reduced in concentration with age, but the majority of the studies so far reported have been concerned with the two enzymes, UDP-galactose transferase which is in part involved in the introduction of a galactose molecule into the proteokeratan molecule, and UDP-glucose transferase which, together with UDP-galactose transferase, is responsible for the introduction of sugar molecules into the hydroxylysine linked glycoproteins of the collagen molecules (Spiro and Spiro, 1971).

The final stage in the synthesis of each individual glycosaminoglycan chain in the proteoglycan, is the introduction of the sulphate. Evidence which has been obtained for alterations in the relative amounts of CS-4, CS-6 and KS proteoglycans in polysaccharide-rich tissues such as cartilage and intervertebral disc (Mathews, 1973) coupled with other evidence for alterations in the rate at which ^{35}S-sulphate is incorporated into the various glycans (Silberberg and Lesker, 1973) demonstrates that different sulphate transferases are responsible for the sulphation of the different carbon atoms. It is also apparent that the activities of CS-4 and CS-6 sulphate transferases are markedly age and tissue dependent.

The aggregation of proteoglycans requires the synthesis of glycoprotein link molecules, and this again provides a site at which age dependent variations in enzymic activity can affect the structure of the molecule as it exists *in vivo*.

Degradation

Collagenases

Collagenases have been defined by Mandl (1961) as being those enzymes which are capable of degrading native collagen at physiological pH and temperature. Theoretically, therefore, this rules out a number of enzymes which are capable of destroying collagenous tissues, either on account of their predilection for modified collagens or because of their preference for a non physiological pH. Some of these, however do warrant consideration, because of the fact that they apparently have an important role to play in the dissolution of tissues at specific periods in the life cycle.

Contrary to the way in which knowledge concerning the elastase/elastin reaction has developed, much of the early work on the reaction between collagenase and its substrate was carried out using enzymes of bacterial origin, little evidence being produced for the existence of mammalian tissue collagenases until the mid sixties. Circumstantial evidence for collagenase activity could be deduced, however, from the appearance of hydroxyproline, either free or in oligopeptide-bound form, in the urine (see below).

Recently mammalian collagenases have been reported for a variety of tissues, which on account of their metabolic degradation might be expected to contain the enzyme. Rheumatoid arthritis is a disease which is prevalent in the elderly although not exclusively confined to this age group. The identification of a collagenase in the hypertrophic synovium which develops in this condition, therefore, although not specifically confirming an age related synthesis of the enzyme, does explain the reason why joint collagen is often heavily degraded in elderly subjects.

Rheumatoid synovial collagenase has properties which relate it to the general group of mammalian tissue collagenolytic enzymes (Evanson *et al.*, 1967; Lazarus *et al.*, 1968; Evanson, 1970). It can be produced in tissue culture, when it passes into the medium in which rheumatoid synovium is incubated. Secretion starts two or three days after the commencement of incubation and reaches its maximum level after five days. The enzyme is a true collagenase, being without effect on casein at neutral pH but does not attack the synthetic peptide Pz-Pro-Leu-Pro-D-Arg-OH which has been specifically devised for the estimation of certain collagenolytic systems. Moreover it has no catheptic activity, being without effect on haemoglobin at low pH.

Bony tissue suffers continuous remodelling *in vivo* and the catabolism of bone matrix might be expected to involve the action of a collagenase. Fullmer and Lazarus (1967) were able to demonstrate collagenase-like activity in the culture medium in which surviving fragments of bone from a variety of species had been incubated, and its existence has been further confirmed by Evanson *et al.* (1970) and Aer and Kivirikko (1969). Again its production may be age dependent *in vivo*.

Granulation tissue invading a wound is another site in the mammalian body in which a collagenase might be deduced to be active. Excess tissue is synthesised and subsequently digested during wound scar remodelling. Collagenases in skin were first identified in healing wounds by Grillo and Gross

(1967) but Eisen *et al.* (1968) and Eisen (1969) have also prepared the enzyme from normal unwounded skin. This enzyme, which appears to attack the substrate at similar points to those at which other collagenases do, is mainly restricted to the upper layers of the dermis, but is not evenly distributed throughout various sites of the body.

The age distribution of these enzymes has not yet been studied in great detail, but it is known that the remodelling of tissues takes place more frequently in the young, up to 35 % of collagen in young rabbit skin, for instance, being degraded before it is incorporated into an insoluble form (Nimni *et al.*, 1967). It might therefore be assumed that since the products of collagenolysis appear more abundantly in the urine of young subjects (p. 152) that the secretion of collagenase by the cells of the connective tissues is restricted to this period of life. However, Hall (1968a) has suggested that the production of collagenase may continue into old age, but that once cross-links are introduced into the collagen macromolecule, fission of main chain peptide linkages no longer results in the production of low molecular weight material which can be excreted from the body, but in the amorphous material to which the generic name pseudoelastin has been given (Fig. 46). This material being no longer susceptible to attack by collagenase, accumulates in all tissues in which the tropocollagen molecules have already been rendered stable by the formation of stable cross-linkages. If this hypothesis is correct, pseudoelastin production will be restricted to those tissues in which the *de novo* synthesis of collagen is minimal after maturity. Full analysis of all tissues of the body will be necessary before this can be provided unequivocally. At present it can be said that pseudoelastin does occur in dermis and vascular tissues for which the turnover, and hence rate of synthesis of new uncross-linked collagen is minimal (Neuberger *et al.*, 1951) and has not been identified in bone matrix in which resynthesis occurs throughout life.

The appearance of hydroxyproline in urine

Isotopic studies on the metabolism of collagen as a whole suggested that the turnover rates of this protein are low compared with those of other proteins (Neuberger *et al.*, 1951). Once it became possible to separate soluble collagens, from the insoluble matrix of collagenous tissues, however, it could be shown that labelled amino acids are rapidly incorporated into the neutral salt soluble fraction (Harkness *et al.*, 1954). Thereafter the label passes into the insoluble fraction and it is difficult to determine the rate at which it finally disappears from this portion of the total collagen. In 1956, however, Ziff *et al.*, showed that patients maintained on a collagen- or gelatin-free diet continued to excrete hydroxyproline into their urine. Since hydroxyproline cannot be synthesised in the body except by the hydroxylation of proline already incorporated in the protocollagen molecule, the fact that an appreciable fraction of the hydroxyproline in the urine is in peptide form must indicate that it is derived from intact collagen by hydrolytic degradation. Lindstedt and Prockop (1961) and Laitinen (1967) from studies of the decay curves of urinary ^{14}C-hydroxyproline, were able to show that the imino acid in the urine was derived from four pools having half lives of 2 h, 17 h, 5 days and 50–300 days. From this it was possible to deduce that part of the newly synthesised collagen is rapidly degraded even before it is secreted by the fibroblast. In young rats this may account for up to 50% of the total urinary hydroxyproline. Once the soluble collagen has been secreted from the cell it becomes progressively cross-linked, and less susceptible to degradation. The amount of collagen which is newly synthesised, and hence represents the fraction which is most susceptible to degradation, decreases with increasing age not only because the molecules become more heavily cross-linked, but also because the rate of synthesis decreases. For instance protocollagen proline levels are reduced with advancing age (Mussini et al., 1957; Heikkinen and Juva, 1968; Uitto et al., 1969). The rate at which hydroxyproline peptides appear in the urine is also reduced in old age, however, by a simultaneous decrease in the rate of degradation (Lindstedt and Prockop, 1961) the effect of which is additive to that of the reduced synthesis.

TABLE 10. Changes in the urinary excretion of hydroxyproline by human subjects with increasing age. Each value is the mean of more than 20 individuals in each group. All values are expressed in terms of mg hydroxyproline/24h.

Age range	Hydroxyproline
0–1 year	37.5
1–5 years	42.5
6–10 years	67.0
11–15 years	122.5
15–21 years	46.0
Adults (over 21 years)	16.5

The hydroxyproline content of the urine rises four-fold from birth to puberty, and then suffers a ten-fold reduction by the time maturity is reached (Table 10). Kivirikko (1970) has pointed out, however, that figures for 24 h urinary output should be normalised by taking into account changes in body mass. To allow for this he records urinary output in terms of bodily surface area, as mg/24 h/m^2, and shows that the apparent prepubertal increase can in the main be ascribed to changes in body size. In fact infants below six months excrete high levels of hydroxyproline per unit surface area of their bodies. This decreases to about one half to two thirds this value during the period from 1 year to 10 years, and then when the rate of growth increases again, in the immediately prepubertal period there is a concomitant 20% increase in hydroxyproline excretion. A high proportion of the hydroxyproline content of the urine of the very young, is in the free form of the imino acid (Woolf and Norman, 1957; Jagenburg, 1959; O'Brien et al., 1960). It is still not clear how this appears in the urine, since there is as yet no known pathway for its synthesis except in the protocollagen molecule. Excessive amounts of free hydroxyproline have also been identified in the urine of subjects with certain recognised pathological conditions. It is possible that the degradative pathways present in the infant and in the pathological subjects contain enzyme systems capable of cleaving linkages on both sides of the hydroxyproline residues in collagen, over and above the normal content of collagenase.

The size corrected values for urinary output do not change markedly after full maturity has been attained, although there is evidence that the overall output may fall in advanced age.

Elastase

Cellular origins. The enzyme elastase was first identified in the pancreas by Balo and Banga (1949) although Ewald had reported similar elastolytic activity as early as 1890. Balo and Banga were looking for a causative agent for the degeneration of elastic fibres and lamellae such as occurs in aortic media during the development of arteriosclerotic lesions. Unless elastase could also be shown to be synthesised by cells in the vessel walls, its action on the medial elastic tissue could only occur if at some stage it was secreted by the pancreas into the circulation.

A considerable amount of apparently contradictory circumstantial evidence has been reported since 1949 concerning the role of the enzyme, especially relating to the question as to whether it is an endocrine or an exocrine factor. Lansing et al. (1953) studying the teleost fish *Lophius piscatorius* in which the Islets of Langerhans are anatomically separated from the acinar cells, were able to demonstrate the localisation of enzyme synthesis in the Islet tissue. Carter (1956) confirmed this by reducing the elastase content of the pancreas by administering cobalt ions which specifically decrease the activity of Islet cells. Hall et al. (1952) had also reported their inability to identify elastase in extracts from the pancreases of human diabetic subjects. It is, however, possible that the preparation which they examined did not contain the enzyme in its active form, but in the form of its zymogen, which can be activated by treatment with trypsin.

Contrary evidence for the exocrine origin of the enzyme was reported by numerous workers. Bartelheimer et al. (1958); Campagnari and Greggia (1959); Cohen et al. (1958); Grant and Robbins (1955); Kokas et al. (1951); Tindel et al. (1962); Rinderknecht et al. (1968) reported elastase in the pancreatic juice of a number of different species including the dog, cat, chicken and man whilst Cohen *et al.* (1958) showed that following the administration of pilocarpine, the elastase content of pancreas decreases at a parallel rate to that of the lipase which is itself of acinar origin. These workers also suggested that Carter's use of cobalt as a specific Islet cell poison left much to be desired as positive proof of the enzyme's endocrine role, since cobalt might merely lower the metabolic rate of the animal as a whole by affecting the thyroid. The observation by Cohen *et al.* (1958) and Tolnay *et al.* (1962) that elastase could be identified in urine, swung the consensus of opinion towards the belief that at some stage elastase must appear in the circulating plasma. Bencosme and Craston (1958) were of the opinion that neither acinar cells nor cells of the Islets are responsible for the elaboration of the enzyme, but they do not rule out the possibility that elastase is produced by the δ cells or by the stroma of the Islets. Even the isolated Islet tissue in *Lophius* is surrounded by a layer of acinar-type cells and this could account for the segregation of elastase in this part of the pancreas, even although it may be preferentially synthesised by cells which are essentially acinar in type. As will be shown later, there is a considerable possibility that certain physiological factors control the role of the enzyme, so that at some periods of life, the major portion passes into the pancreatic juice, whereas at other times it is secreted into the circulation.

Elastase in the plasma. Although the original concept that elastase was involved in the degradation of the elastic tissue in the artery wall, (Balo and and Banga, 1949) necessitated the passage of elastase through the plasma *en route* from the pancreas, no direct evidence for this was available until 1966. Elastase is accompanied in the plasma, by at least one specific and other nonspecific inhibitors, and these preclude the use of the normal methods for the estimation of the enzyme. Hall (1966), however, demonstrated that it was possible to employ a modified form of elastin as substrate which provided a system which was independent of the presence of the inhibitor. Elastin which has been dyed with Congo-Red not only retains its susceptibility to elastase, but provides a substrate which is twenty times more susceptible than the unstained protein. As the substrate passes into solution under the action of the enzyme, the dye is released into solution and its concentration can be measured at a wavelength of 485 nm. Banga and Ardelt (1967) and Geokas *et al.* (1968) have criticised the method on account of the fact that Congo-Red has a high affinity for albumin and hence that the liberation of dye from the stained substrate by plasma or serum may reflect its interaction with albumin and may not necessarily be a function of enzymic activity at all. This point was, however, fully dealt with by Hall in his original paper. A correct choice of the relative amounts of substrate and plasma permits the elimination of any physicochemical effect due to the albumin content of the plasma. If the amount of plasma added is raised so as to increase the potential amount of enzyme to be estimated, the initial linearity of the response curve is lost, presumably due to the involvement of the albumin fraction. Below this cut-off level of 5 μl/10 μg Congo-Red-dyed elastin, the effect is essentially due to the enzyme alone. Confirmation of this has recently been obtained by the observation (Hall and El-Ridi, 1976a, b) that elastase which will react with both unstained and Congo-Red-dyed elastin can be isolated from plasma by electrofocusing.

Hall (1968b) examined the elastase levels of plasmas from human subjects of various age groups ranging from birth to 90 years of age (Figs 63 and 64). A considerable scatter was observed, but the overall pattern for this group was identical with that observed later for a completely different population (Hall, 1973b) and showed marked differences between males and females. Elastase levels can be quantified in terms of E.units/ml (Hall and El-Ridi, 1976a, b), but since there is still little standardisation in the methods used to obtain the fundamental elastin substrate from which the Congo-Red-dyed elastin is prepared, Hall has usually recorded enzymic activity in terms of arbitrary figures which are comparative over the whole age range, but which are not necessarily directly comparable at an absolute level with those reported by other workers.

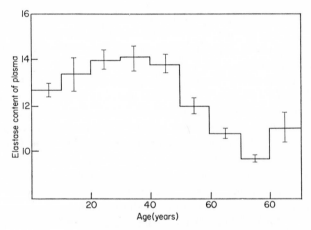

FIG. 63. The elastase content of plasma for male subjects grouped in 5 year age groups. The vertical bar in each step indicates the standard deviation of each five year mean. The values quoted are arbitrary assessments of elastase activity. This applies to Figs 64, 65 and 66.

The values for elastase activity in male plasma rise by 10% over the period from birth to 25 years of age, and subsequently fall to a lowest level at 80.

There is a slight rise thereafter, but this may be due to natural selection among survivors to this advanced age, and should not necessarily be taken as indicating a true upsurge in elastase content as a direct result of age. Values for the levels of elastase activity in female plasma appear to fall steadily with age except for a period between 50 and 60, when the elastase content lies considerably above the general level. Tesal and Hall (1972) have pointed out that

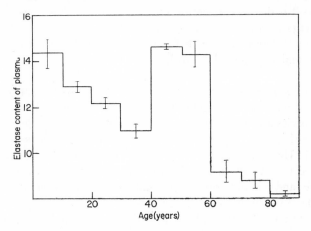

FIG. 64. The elastase content of plasma from female subjects expressed as in Fig. 63.

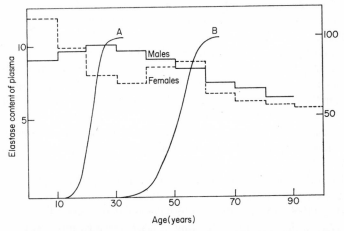

FIG. 65. The comparison of peak activity of male and female plasma elastase with the periods, represented by the lines A and B respectively, when androgen secretion is either assuming its greatest level during the onset of male sexual maturity (line A) or is uncontrolled by the simultaneous secretion of oestrogens during the menopause (line B).

the appearance of peak levels of elastase in both male and female plasma follows shortly after that stage in hormonal development at which androgen secretion is at its maximum. Androgen secretion in the male increases over the immediately post-pubertal period to reach a maximum at sexual maturity. This rise is shortly followed by a point of maximum appearance of elastase in the plasma (Fig. 65). Androgen secretion, uncomplicated by the simultaneous presence of oestrogens, is at its greatest at the menopause in the female, and it is during this period of life that the highest concentration of elastase occurs in the female plasma. The reason for this has not yet been elucidated but it would appear that the appearance of elastase in the plasma is probably under hormonal control.

Elastase content of the pancreas. Loeven (1960, 1967) has isolated two forms of elastoproteinase from pig and human pancreases, and Hall has shown that these two species are similar in structure and activity to the calcium-poor (E) and calcium-rich (ECa) forms isolated by completely different methods (Hall, 1970a, 1971; Hall and Tesal, 1976) (see p. 133). Loeven reported that the amount of E rose nearly three-fold in the male pancreases during the first 40 years of life, and fell away rapidly to a constant low level thereafter. ECa on the other hand which was on average present at between two and five times the concentration of E throughout the whole of the life span, reached its highest level at between 30 and 40 years of age, and then also fell away, but at a slower rate than that at which the levels of E declined. Female pancreases contained significantly less of both forms of enzyme throughout life, and the amount of the dimeric ECa form of the enzyme was especially low in the sixth decade, E was also very low in subjects of this age, but the levels in other age groups were not sufficiently high for differences to be significant.

The fact that Leoven observed very low levels of enzyme in the pancreases of females at exactly the same period of life when high concentrations are apparent in the plasma, may provide definite evidence in favour of a hormonal regulation of elastase synthesis and secretion.

The appearance of a given concentration of enzyme in the plasma depends on three factors which are simultaneously effective. Firstly on the rate of synthesis of the enzyme in the cells of the organ concerned. Secondly on its release from the cells into the plasma, and lastly on systems which destroy or adsorb the enzyme, thus effectively removing it from the circulation. Gore and Larkey (1960) and Loeven (1969) have isolated elastase from the tissues of the artery wall, thus demonstrating at least one way in which the third of these factors could operate. The amounts of enzyme present in the pancreas on the one hand, and in the plasma on the other, reflect the simultaneous operation of the other two. Since the method of analysis which is based on the use of Congo-Red-dyed elastin and substrate does not distinguish between the two forms of the enzyme, it is most appropriate to compare the plasma levels, and low levels in the tissue. It appears therefore that the rates of both synthesis and secretion vary throughout life, and since in both sexes secretion appears to be maximal during periods of imbalance or active secretion of androgenic hormones, it would appear that it is this which may control one or other or both of these phenomena.

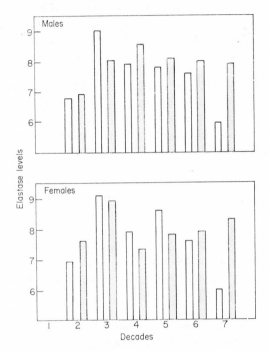

FIG. 66. The effect of pseudoxanthoma elasticum on plasma elastase levels. The open columns are age matched normal subjects (a different population to that referred to in Figs 63 and 64); the black columns represent subjects with frank clinical signs of PXE.

Hall (1973b) reported age changes which differ from those of the normal ones quoted above, in the levels of elastase present in the plasma of subjects suffering from the hereditary connective tissue disease, pseudoxathoma elasticum. In this study unaffected male and female relatives of those with the disease were used as controls. Once again the normal female peri-menopausal group showed elevated plasma levels, followed by a reduction in subsequent decades (Fig. 66). The rise between the fourth and fifth decade was not, however, followed by a fall, in the case of individuals with the disease, and the elastase level of the 70+ group was virtually as high as that of the plasma of the 20–30-year old group. The elastase content of plasma from male subjects with clinical signs of pseudoxanthoma elasticum only fell by 9% between the fourth and seventh decades, whereas the elastase content of the plasma of the control population fell by 22% over the same period.

Pseudoxanthoma elasticum is characterised by dermatological, ophthalmalogical, gastrointestinal and haematological symptoms together with the involvement of the peripheral vascular tissues which include arterial, venous, cardiac, cerebrovascular and hypertensvie complications. Although all these symptoms are now recognised as being part of a single syndrome (Pope, 1972), they do not necessarily stem from the same basic biochemical lesion. McKusick (1966), however, has recorded elastic degeneration in the coronary vessels and aneurysms in patients with pseudoxanthoma, whilst haematemeses have been observed by a number of workers, (Holmes-Spicer, 1919; von Tannerheim, 1901; Carlborg, 1944; Eddy and Farber, 1962) presumably due to elastic degeneration such as that reported by Flatley et al. (1963). When these findings are taken in conjunction with the observations of altered dermal elastin, which are universal in pseudoxanthoma, it is not surprising that differences in plasma elastase levels occur between those with the disease and the controls. In these studies, the marked variation from normal which occurs at all ages above the third decade provides an interesting subject for further consideration, since there does not appear to be any clinical evidence for the disease to be more prevalent in older age groups.

Loeven and Baldwin (1971a) have studied elastase levels in the pancreases of rats, and have demonstrated a marked increase between 15 and 18 months of age. It is not yet apparent how this observation can be related to the observations of human pancreases.

Elastase inhibitor. In addition to inhibition by relatively high concentrations of various salts (Lewis et al., 1956; Winter and Frankel, 1956; Tolnay and Bagdy, 1959; Thomas and Partridge, 1960; Amati and Castelli, 1961; Lamy et al., 1961; Hall, 1964) and by chelating agents (Hall, 1954, 1961b, 1970b) there is considerable evidence for the control of elastolysis by an inhibitor present in the plasma.

Balo and Banga (1955); Robert and Samuel (1957) and Walford and Schneider (1959) separated an inhibitor from serum, and identified it as being associated with the a_1-globulin fraction. Graham (1958) observed two inhibitory fractions in serum, and suggested that one was specific for elastase with a lesser degree of cross-specificity for trypsin, whereas the other was mainly a trypsin inhibitor with a secondary effect on elastase. Loeven and Baldwin (1971b) have examined the elastase and trypsin inhibitors in rat plasma, and their dissimilarity can be deduced from the fact that whereas the amount of trypsin inhibitor in rat plasma falls with increasing age at a rate of 2% per month over the period from birth to 17 months, the elastase inhibitor level rises by 1.8% per month over the same period (Fig. 67). The two inhibitors are therefore, completely separate entities, and any cross reaction which may occur, must be due to a fundamental similarity of the reactive centres of the two enzymes themselves, and not to the molecular identity of the inhibitors.

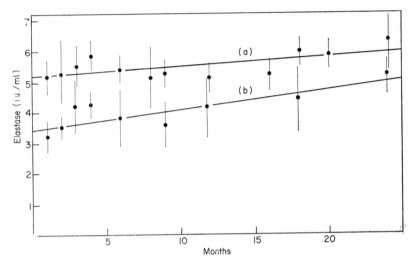

FIG. 67. Elastase inhibitor levels in male (a) and female (b) rat plasma.

Walford and Schneider (1959) measured the amounts of elastase inhibitor present in the sera of various animals and showed that the effect of small amounts of serum up to 1 μl/10 μg elastase (Hall, 1962) produced between 85% inhibition of elastolysis in the case of mouse serum and 28% for dog serum. With human serum the value is in between at 56 and 66% for males and females respectively. Graham (1958) reported lower levels (a mean value of 38%) and this was confirmed by Hall (1966) who recorded values ranging from 28 to 50%. Contrary to the observations of Walford and Schneider, he also reported the existence of marked age variations. A significant increase is apparent in the amounts of inhibitor present in the plasma of both male and female groups during the first 30 to 40 years of life ($p = 0.05$ for males and 0.025 for females) followed by a slow decrease over the next 40 years ($p = 0.025$ and 0.028 respectively). Both male and female subjects of ages above 60 demonstrated higher levels of inhibitor than the 60-year old groups (Fig. 68). The relatively small number of males made it impossible to determine whether this rise was significant or not, but the rise in the case of the larger female group was highly significant ($p = 0.005$). This may represent an overall elevant in the inhibitor levels of all individuals at ages above 60, but since these studies were of necessity cross-sectional and not longitudinal, may more likely represent the survival of a subgroup which throughout life had provided the upper portion of the distribution of elastase inhibitor levels, just as has been suggested for the similar rise which occurs in the plasma elastase levels at advanced age.

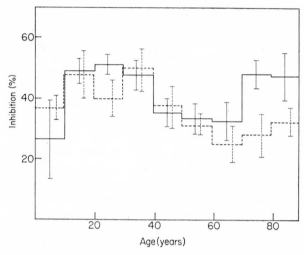

Fig. 68. The percentage inhibition of a standard elastase system induced by the addition of 5 μl plasma. The population was identical to that for which elastase levels are reported in Figs 63 and 64. (Unbroken line, females; dashed line, males).

Of the group studied by Hall (1966), 8.5% had no inhibitor at all in their plasma; in fact the addition of their plasma to a reaction mixture already containing elastase induced a degree of elastolysis which was higher than that produced by the added elastase alone, thus confirming the existence of elastase in the plasma. Of those subjects with elastase inhibitor in their plasma and for whom elastase levels could be measured by the use of Congo-Red-dyed elastin as substrate (Hall, 1966) an inverse relationship between enzyme and inhibitor levels could be demonstrated. This indicates that inhibitor production is not induced in direct response to the presence of elastase.

Age-related variations in elastase inhibitor in rat plasma (Loeven and Baldwin, 1971b) do not coincide with those observed in human plasma. The rat inhibitor rises in a roughly linear fashion (r = 0.45) for the whole period from birth to two years of age. This may indicate that the production of the inhibitor is controlled in a different fashion in rats from that which is operative in man. It may, however, indicate that the rate at which a rat population ages is different from that for human subjects since in the few female rats studied by Loeven and Baldwin a rapid fall could be observed at ages above

2 years. It may, therefore, be that at least as far as the appearance of elastase inhibitor in the plasma is concerned, the period of two years during which the inhibitor level increases is comparable to the period of the human life span up to 40 years of age during which the inhibitor level rises in human plasma also.

Proteoglycanases

The integrity of the glycosaminoglycan fraction in connective tissue is maintained by the simultaneous activity of synthetic and degradative enzyme systems, just as is the case with the protein constituents. The intact proteo-glycan or proteoglycan aggregate with its glycosaminoglycan, protein and link glycoprotein elements is subject to attack by a large number of enzymes with a variety of functions. The protein backbone itself may be degraded by a variety of proteolytic systems of which pronase and papain, although not endogenous have proved of most use in the study of the structure of these complex molecules. Proteolytic enzymes of suitable activity for the fission of main chain peptide linkages in the protein fraction of the proteoglycan mole-cules, are present in various tissues (Barrett and Dingle, 1971) many of them being derived from lysosomes within the connective tissue cells. Cathepsins B1 and D are the most likely to effect large scale degradation of the protein fraction, although they do so to different degrees; exhaustive treatment with Cathepsin D resulting in degradation products of much higher molecular weight than are produced by similar treatment with Cathepsin B1 (Morrison, 1970).

The linkage between each glycosaminoglycan chain and the protein core could theoretically be cleaved by a β-xylosidase, since it consists of a xylosyl O-serine bond. β-xylosidase is, however, without effect on intact proteochondro-glycan, and it appears that if the complete separation of protein and glyco-saminoglycan or their degradation products occurs at any point in the degradation of the whole macro-molecule, it can only do so after one or other component has been degraded. This would presumably minimise any steric effects which prevent the enzyme reaching the root of the side chain.

Linkages within the length of the glycosaminoglycan side chains are hydro-lysed by one or other of a group of glycolytic enzymes specific for the 1–3 or 1–4 linkages which exist between galatose or glucuronic acid and N-acetyl-glucosamine, such as β-galactosidase, β-glucoronidase, or N-acetylgusoamini-dase, whereas the presence of an α-glycosidically linked L-iduronic acid in dermatan sulphate would indicate that an α-L-iduronidase is required for the complete degradation of this polysaccharide. All these enzymes have been identified in one or other of the tissues in which their specific substrates occur. It is not as yet clear whether the changing ratios of CS and KS chains in cartilage proteoglycan are dependent on varying degrees of synthesis of one or other of these components, coupled with a constant rate of degradation, i.e. the presence of a constant level of the appropriate glycolytic enzyme, or conversely due to a constant rate of synthesis coupled with changing digestive activity.

A further reaction which is under enzymic control is the removal of the sulphate residue from the polysaccharide. There is an appreciable amount of evidence which demonstrates that the removal of sulphate from chondroitin and from dermatan chains is accomplished by different enzymes (Buddecke and Kresse, 1974).

Silberberg and Lesker (1973) have shown that the amounts of β-glucoronidase and β-galactosidase present in the lysosomes of guinea pig articular cartilage rise with age from 12 weeks to $2\frac{1}{2}$ years. There are slight reductions in both enzymes at earlier ages, but the glucuronidase activity increases eleven-fold from 0.5 μmoles/gDNA/h at 12 weeks to 5.5. μmoles/gDNA/h at $2\frac{1}{2}$ years and the galactosidase from 0.75 μmoles/h to 3 μmoles/h. After $2\frac{1}{2}$ years the level of glucuronidase falls rapidly, whereas the galactosidase activity increases at a reduced rate. Over the same period of adult life sulphatose activity of the same tissue, increases in line with the glucuronidase, but during the period of advancing senility from $2\frac{1}{2}$ years to $5\frac{1}{2}$ years, it mirrors more closely the changes observed in the galactosidase. Davidson and Woodhall (1959) have reported that similar changes resulting in the degradation of the glycosaminoglycans of the intervertebral disc occur with increasing age.

Lipolytic systems

The concept that some at least of the lipids which are present in connective tissue are firmly bound to the protein constituents is not a new one. Lansing (1954a, 1959) and Labella (1957) referred to elastin as a metabolically active lipoprotein, and Saxl and Hall (1967) and Saxl (1961) produced evidence for the interaction of elastin proteins with lipid to form a firmly bound complex. Melcher (1969) identified lipid association with other components of connective tissues, and Maggi *et al.* (1964) differentiated between free and bound lipids in tissues. Once it has been accepted that lipids form an integral part of certain individual connective tissue components, it becomes necessary to look for lipolytic enzyme systems which may be involved in the removal and hydrolysis of such lipid during the degradation of connective tissue, either as a result of the ageing process itself, or of one of the age dependent pathological conditions which affect this type of tissue.

Early studies of elastolysis were based on Balo's search for an agent which could be involved in the development of atherosclerotic lesions. Since two of the factors observed in the development of the artery wall lesion were reduplication of the internal elastic lamina and lipid deposition, and it was possible that they might be in some way related, it was natural that attempts were made to utilise preparations of elastase which might be capable of reducing the apparent elastosis of the intimal region of the aorta to eliminate more than one aspect of the syndrome. Lansing (1954a) and Szabo and Cseh (1962) suggested that elastase had lipolytic activity, and Butturini *et al.* (1959a, b, c); Citi *et al.* (1960) and Lapiccirella *et al.* (1960a, b) reported the prevention of lipid deposition and a reduction in circulating cholesterol in the plasma of chickens and other animals fed diets rich in cholesterol.

Hall (1953) first suggested that elastase as extracted from pancreatic tissue was not unitary in nature, and this was confirmed when elastomucase was separated from enzymes with true elastolytic activity (Hall, 1956, 1958; Loeven, 1963). Hall (1967); Saxl and Hall (1967) and Saxl (1957b) were initially of the opinion that the apparent lipolytic activity of crude elastase preparations was due to the release of a polysaccharide, believed to react in a similar fashion to heparin in activating a lipoprotein lipase type enzyme which had the effect of preventing the deposition of lipid in the artery wall and lowering the level of lipid in the circulation. Loeven (1964), however, was able to demonstrate a separate enzyme, lipoprotein lipase in the pancreas. Later Miller *et al.* (1970); Miller (1971); Teale (1971) and Teale *et al.* (1972) isolated enzyme systems from pancreas in fractions which in their crude form contained both elastase and elastomucase, which were capable of hydrolysing both free triglyceride and lipoprotein triglyceride, and also hydrolysing and synthesising ester linkages with cholesterol.

The age dependence of these latter enzymes has not yet been studied in detail, but there is considerable evidence for age changes in the amounts of elastolipoproteinase in the pancreas and the circulation.

Loeven (1963, 1965a) extending the earlier observations of Hall (1958) used the synergistic effects of the nonproteolytic members of the elastase complex of enzymes to identify them in the α-globulin fraction of plasma. Hall (1958) had shown that when certain fractions separated by paper electrophoresis from crude pancreatic extracts were added to pure preparations of elastase, the total activity, measured in terms of protein dissolved, was greater than the sum of the activities of the two enzymes tested separately. The addition of the fraction to which the name elastomucase was given, also brought more polysaccharide into solution, whereas the simultaneous presence of the elastolipoproteinase fraction resulted in the release of fatty acids from the elastic tissue. Loeven (1967) eluted elastolytic enzymes from DEAE-Sephadex with a step-wise salt gradient, in a pH 8.8 bicarbonate-HCl buffer, and indentified elastolipoproteinase activity in the fraction eluting in 0.1M sodium chloride.

Loeven (1969) was unable to identify elastolipoproteinase in extracts of the aortic wall of either young or old cattle.

Hormonal control of connective tissue metabolism

Chalones

When a wound is made through the skin, severing both epidermis and the deeper layers of the dermis, growth of dermis to fill the wound occurs quite rapidly and ceases when the required amount of tissue has been provided. For many years it was believed that such growth was induced by a *positive* feedback mechanism activating the fibroblasts in the region of the wound and being switched off as soon as the wound had healed. No such hormone has ever been identified, and over recent years studies have tended towards the opposite concept that tissue mass is controlled by *negative* feed-back. Thus Mercer (1962) on purely theoretical grounds suggested that the thickness of the epidermis could be controlled by a factor, the synthesis of which was proportional to the epidermal thickness, which inhibited the mitosis of epidermal cells. Bullough and Laurence (1960a, b) confirmed this by extraction of a glycoprotein with a molecular weight of about 30 000 which selectively inhibits epidermal mitotic activity (Bullough *et al.*, 1964; Hondius-Boldingh and Laurence, 1968) to which the generic term chalone has been applied. Bullough and Laurence (1960b) and Houck (1971) have produced evidence that dermal fibroblasts and other connective tissue cells release inhibitor substances.

Chalones vary considerably in size and nature, ranging in molecular weight from 4000 to 50 000 daltons. Although some are glycopeptide or glycoprotein in nature, others are essentially protein in composition. They appear to be synthesised continuously within tissue cells and continuously secreted by the cells into the extracellular space, where they appear to be degraded, although Bullough and Laurence (1971) have identified active chalones in blood and urine, thus indicating that they may have a relatively long half life in the organism.

Although the concept of chalones was introduced to explain the control of organ size by actively mitotic cells, it has also been demonstrated that they are able to react with post-mitotic cells, where they control the rate of ageing of these elements. Thus a burst of mitotic activity such as accompanies the removal of tissue in a wound, will result in an acceleration of the ageing, and a hastening of the ultimate death of these post-mitotic cells in the area, which come under the control of the specific chalones released by the cells surrounding the wound (Bullough, 1973).

The activity of chalones although ubiquitous in the cellular components of all tissues, may not represent the whole of the mitotic-control mechanism. Bullough (1967) has shown for instance that the diurnal mitotic cycle may be the result of the interaction or simultaneous action of chalones and two stress hormones, adrenaline and an as yet uncharacterised glucocorticosteroid. Thus a reduction in the out-pouring of such stress hormones during sleep results in a failure to maintain repression of mitosis, and hence in tissue proliferation, whereas on waking the combined activity of stress hormone and chalone reduce mitosis, thus preventing tissue growth. ACTH and adrenal corticoids have also been shown to delay the formation of granulation tissue in wounds, and this may probably be due to similar activation of a chalone effect (Kendall *et al.*, 1949).

Anabolic steroids

Directly opposite effects to those attributed to the stress hormones can be ascribed to hormones such as testosterone, which have anabolic character-istics. Various effects have been reported, but the diversity of result would appear to be dependent on the nutritional status of the animal. Thus Tauben-haus and Amromin (1950) noted impaired formation of granulation tissue around a turpentine induced abscess following testosterone treatment of animals maintained on a protein deficient diet, whereas Loddi and Maggi (1953) observed an increase in the tensile strength of a healing skin wound following testosterone treatment of a fully fed animal. Pearce *et al.* (1960), however, could find no change in the healing wounds of rats fed a normal diet. Viljanto *et al.* (1962) on the other hand observed increases in hydroxy-proline concentration and tensile strength in wound repair tissue in rats after treatment with anabolic steroids.

Studies on the effects of anabolic steroids on the individual components of connective tissues stem from observations on the glycosaminoglycan content of sexual tissues such as the cock's comb (Ludwig *et al.*, 1950). The effect of testosterone, however, is not restricted to tissues such as this which may be regarded as its major target organ. Allalauf and Ber (1961) have reported that the systemic administration of testosterone results in an accumulation of uronic acid in the skin of the rat. Kowaleski (1957, 1958a, b) has shown that 17-ethyl-19-nortestosterone, but neither methyl testosterone nor testosterone propionate, stimulates the uptake of ^{35}S-sulphate into the glycosaminoglycans of the growing bones of young cockerels and of the callouses which form in the repair of fractured humeri. From these studies and those of Huble (1957) and Salmon *et al.* (1963) it may be deduced that the synthesis of sulphated glyco-saminoglycans is under hormonal control. Since these polysaccharides control the synthesis of collagen fibrils, it therefore appears that the synthesis of the collagenous component of connective tissue is itself also under hormonal control. Although part at least of the tensile properties of a connective tissue are directly dependent on the GAG content, the major structural component is the collagen fibre, and hence if collagen synthesis is not directly under hormonal control, the indirect effect via the glycosaminoglycan has an equally important role to fulfil.

The development of the cock's comb is an age-dependent phenomenon, being determined by the increased secretion of testosterone by the Leydig cells of the testis under the control of gonadotrophin. 17-Hydroxycorticosteroid excretion in the urine, may not be unequivocally indicative of similar levels in the circulation, but will certainly be related to its rise from 2 mg/24 h at 5 years of age to 20 mg by full maturity, and the slow fall to 3–12 mg in senility. The consequent changes in glycosaminoglycan content in the connective tissues can easily be observed.

Thyroid hormone

L-Thyroxine by itself brings about a reduction in the concentration of both hexosamine and hydroxyproline in connective tissue such as the wall of the aorta, but when administered in association with adrenaline, the effect is completely different. Lorenzen (1959, 1962) has shown that the total dry weights of rabbit aortas, and their hexosamine, uronic acid and hydroxyproline contents increase significantly after 12 days injection of a mixture of L-thyroxine and adrenaline. One group of Lorenzen's animals which were killed 14 days subsequently showed abnormal values for all these parameters, but all the other groups of animals sacrificed 3, 7, 21 and 28 days after the cessation of hormone therapy showed nearly two- and one half-fold increases in total dry weight, uronic acid and hydroxyproline and a nearly three-fold increase in hexosamine.

The thyroid gland suffers progressive atrophy with increasing age and Pittman (1962) and Good (1958) suggested that ageing is due to this slowly developing hypofunction. However, the thyroid reacts equally to stimulation by thyroid stimulating hormone (TSH) (Baker et al., 1959) in both young and old. Hence it would appear most likely that any reduction in thyroid activity and hence in thyroid-induced alterations in connective tissue metabolism, may be due to a failure of the pituitary to produce TSH. Lederer and Bataille (1969), however, were able to note sub-optimal responses to TSH in the elderly. Whether the ultimate point of control lies in the thyroid or the pituitary, there is at least one age-related change which can be shown to be under hormonal control, and which under certain conditions comes under the influence of the thyroid. The vocal cords change their fundamental resonance under the influence of the male sex hormones. Leutert (1964) has recorded the type of change which can be associated with age. The collagen content of the vocal cords increases in the male at puberty, whilst in the female at the same stage of development there is a massive increase in elastic tissue. With increasing age the collagen bundles show increasing numbers of regions of localised necrosis. The gruff voice associated with myxoedema may well be associated with a reduction in the tone of the vocal cords, due to a failure to synthesise new tissue to replace those components which are suffering the normal degree of catabolic remodelling.

Oestrogens

Female sex hormones control tissue growth, as can easily be observed from the marked morphological changes which accompany the attainment of menarche and the cessation of menstruation at the menopause. Oestrogenic hormones are produced in increasing amounts in girls between 10 and 17 years of age, and appear in the urine in increasing amounts over this period, rising from below 1 μg/24 h to between 13 and 56 μg/24 h at various times during the fully operative menstrual cycle. At the climacteric the level of oestrogen in the urine may fall to as low as 5 μg/24 h, indicating a marked reduction in the circulating level of the hormone. The development of the breasts, and the remodelling of the skeleton which accompany the biochemical pubertal changes are in part brought about by the anabolic activities of the oestrogens on connective tissues of these regions of the body. The atrophy which occurs in a number of tissues following the menopause, is indirectly due to the action of the oestrogens since the anabolic effects of these substances are no longer adequate to offset the catabolic activity which is still retained. The major changes which have been shown to accompany the menopause are thinning skin (McConkey *et al.*, 1963) and osteoporosis (McConkey *et al.*, 1965) in both instances being apparently due to a failure to synthesise new collagen. Post and pre-menopausal treatment with oestrogens (Henneman and Wallack, 1957) interferes with the loss of bone which accompanies the menopause, as can be seen from the fact that subjects already showing signs of osteoporosis and its associated reduction in stature, either remain at the same height or soon stabilise and suffer no further loss of height, immediately after oestrogen therapy.

Oestrogens are also involved in the repression of the metabolism of elastin. Gilfillan *et al.* (1960, 1961); Schneider *et al.* (1960) and Walford and Sopher (1966) have reported the occurrence of marked increases in the levels of the plasma inhibitor for elastase during pregnancy. When these observations are considered alongside the fact that androgens appear to control the secretion and activity of the enzyme itself, it would appear that the oestrogen/androgen balance may be of considerable importance in maintaining the level of elastin in the connective tissues of the body.

The pituitary. Direct experimentation on the effect of the pituitary hormones on the ageing of connective tissue has not proved easy to perform. A certain amount of research has been carried out on one or two of the trophic hormones. This will be dealt with below, after the effects of total hypophysectomy have been considered.

The long term effect of hypophysectomy is a retardation of the ageing of collagen. This has been demonstrated (Everitt and Olsen, 1965) by studies of the breaking time of collagen fibres after immersion in 7M urea solution

(Elden and Boucek, 1962). Verzar and Spichtin (1966) measured the tension induced in rat tail tendons on thermal denaturation in animals aged $4\frac{1}{2}$ to 24 months, which had been hypophysectomised at $1\frac{1}{2}$ months. At all ages the tension in the tendons of hypophysectomised animals was less than 90% of that of normal animals of the same age. The mean value for the ratio of 32 pairs of animals over the whole age range was 73% indicating that on average the ageing of the rat tail is retarded by about 30% by hypophysectomy. Verzar and Spichtin (1966) also showed that the "labile" fraction of collagen, i.e. that fraction which dissolves in Ringer's solution in 10 min at 60 °C (Verzar and Meyer, 1959) is approximately 50% higher in dorsal skin of hypophysectomised animals than in their paired controls (Fig. 69). The rate at which the labile fraction decreases with age is the same for both groups of animals, thus indicating that ageing still continues after the removal of the pituitary, but from the fact that the level for hypophysectomised animals is higher throughout, it can be implied that the ageing process is retarded considerably.

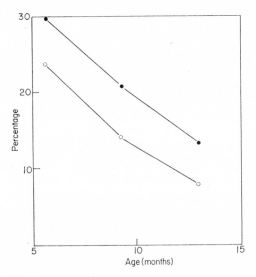

FIG. 69. The amounts of labile collagen in the dorsal skin of normal (○) and hypophysectionised (●) rats, over the age range 6 to 13 months (after Verzar and Spichtin, 1966).

Whether the involvement of the pituitary in this ageing phenomenon has been proved unequivocally, is however, still in doubt, since hypophysectomy has been shown to reduce appetite and Everitt (1971) has shown that the growth and ageing of tail tendon collagen is dependent on food intake.

Catabolic hormones. The physiological and biochemical activities of para-thormone have been under investigation for some number of years. The administration of the hormone to normal subjects and those with hypopara-thyroidism regularly increases the excretion of hydroxyproline into the urine (Avioli *et al.*, 1966; Keiser *et al.*, 1964). Since the level of urinary hydroxy-proline is greatest during periods of massive collagen synthesis these observa-tions could indicate either that parathormone was activating the fibroblastic synthesis of collagen or conversely activating the secretion of collagenase by the tissue cells. Tammes (1964) was unable to demonstrate any effect on the administration of parathormone to cultures of chick lung tissue, whereas Walker *et al.* (1964) and Harris and Sjoerdsma (1966) observed the stimu-lation of collagenase synthesis, and the resorption of collagen *in vivo*. It has not yet been demonstrated that senile osteoporosis is directly associated with the activity of the parathyroid glands. In fact hypoparathyroidism is usually an infantile condition, and hyperparathyroidism is nearly always of malignant origin. However, the former, when apparent in adults is often associated with lenticular cataracts, hence it may have some temporal signifi-cance.

Adenomas of the adrenal cortex presenting as Cushing's Syndrome, result in a number of symptoms which may be related to changes in the connective tissues. The skin is universally thinner, there is also bruising due to loss of skin tone, poor wound healing and a variety of lesions in the vascular tissue. Here again there is little evidence for the onset of Cushing's Syndrome being age dependent except for the fact that adenomas in general develop in the period 25–40. However, synthetic steroids closely related to those produced naturally by the adrenal cortex are frequently administered to subjects of advancing years and this has permitted studies to be made on the effects of such substances on connective tissue metabolism over a wide age range.

Cortisone, hydrocortisone, prednisolone and dexamethasone are often ad-ministered as anti-inflammatory agents in rheumatoid and arthritic conditions. Hall *et al.* (1974) studied the collagen content of skin samples from the midline of the thigh in control subjects and patients to whom prednisolone had been administered. The collagen content of the dermis expressed as μg collagen/mm^2 of skin surface and representing the total amount in a column of skin from epidermis through to the sub-dermal faschia, fell in normal female sub-jects from 280 μg/mm^2 at age 30 to 180 at age 90. Similar figures for subjects receiving prednisolone therapy were 220 and 120. Thus, although the rates of collagen loss with age were identical at about 1.4 μg/mm^2/year, the predniso-lone treated subjects invariably had 22% less collagen than the controls. The nature of the collagen in the skin could be seen from a study of the amount of soluble collagen present. Whereas the soluble collagen content of the nor-mal skins fell with age in agreement with previous observations by Jackson and Bentley (1968); Bakerman (1964), etc., the soluble collagen content of skin samples from prednisolone treated subjects was 37% higher in a 57–78 year age group than in a 20–56 year age group. These observations are cross-sectional and hence subject to individual variation. However, a small number of subjects were re-examined after 1 year's treatment with prednisolone when it was observed that the amount of collagen lost, following treatment with the steroid, was directly proportional to the age of the subject (Fig. 70), rising from 30 μg/mm²/year at 30 years of age to 130 μg/mm²/year at 80. There did not appear to be any direct correlation between the amount of collagen lost and the dose of prednisolone administered. Presumably there is a threshold level above which this catabolic effect is apparent.

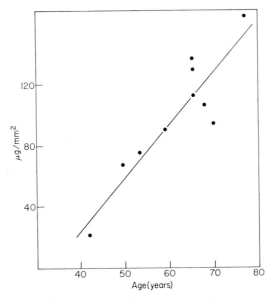

FIG. 70. The relationship of the loss of collagen (soluble and insoluble) from the skins of female subjects with rheumatoid arthritis, during 12 months treatment with prednisolone, to their age at the commencement of the treatment.

Vogel (1974) reported a 74% decrease in skin thickness in rats treated for 60 days with 10 or 25 mg cortisol/kg body weight. This loss was quite comparable with loss of total body weight which was 76% over the same period. The ultimate load at rupture of these skin samples fell by 62% over this period, but on account of the reduction in skin thickness the tensile strength rose from 113.7 kp/cm² to 167.5 kp/cm² over this period of cortisol treatment. The proportion of insoluble collagen to the total collagen content of the skin rose from 7.44 to 11.57. Although this was in part due to an increase in the absolute amount of the collagen which was in the insoluble form, it was dependent to a certain extent on a reduction in the amount of collagen which was resistant to extraction by 0.15M NaCl, but could be removed from the tissue by 0.5M NaCl. This fraction represents the newly synthesised tropocollagen molecules which have, however, already been incorporated into the microfibrillar structure. Neither the easily extractable, i.e. very recently synthesised collagen, nor the citrate soluble material which represents collagen which is fully incorporated into the microfibrillar fraction were markedly affected by cortisol treatment. Shorter periods of cortisol treatment (5 days) resulted in a reduction in synthesis with proportionally greater amounts of collagen appearing in the more highly organised fractions. Contrary to the observations of human skin (Hall *et al.*, 1974) there was a progressively greater effect the larger the dose of steroid.

Vogel (1974) does not give details of the ages of the rats employed for this study, but in view of the fact that the group of control rats for the 5 day treatment with cortisol weighed 150 g whereas the controls for the 60 day experiment weighed 382 g, it may be deduced that the former were being treated during a period of growth, whereas the treatment period for the latter group spanned both growth and maturation, probably extending minimally into the senile period. It is not possible to determine how closely these observations are in agreement with those on human skin, since the periods of treatment of Vogel's rat experiments overlap. However, if the results obtained in this study are converted to conform to total skin collagen loss per unit surface area, it can be seen that the 60 day treatment with cortisol results in an increase in collagen content which is 3.7 times greater than that which is induced by 5 days' treatment. It would, therefore, appear very unlikely that an age-dependent reduction in collagen content such as is reported for human skin can occur in the skin of old rats.

6

Age-Dependent Pathological Conditions in Connective Tissues

One of the difficulties which has been associated throughout with all studies of the ageing process, has been the inability on the part of the research workers concerned to disentangle the truly physiological phenomena from those which could only be regarded as being of pathological origin. Some pathological situations, such as infection by external organisms, might on the face of it appear easy to classify, but one of the parameters by which ageing may be assessed must be the extent to which older members of a population are unable to respond favourably to non-physiological stress in the way that they were able to during early adulthood. The stress may be endogenous, or introduced from outside the organism itself. Therefore, even infection, or at least the body's changing response to infection may justifiably be considered in studies of the ageing process.

Some workers (Craciun, 1973) have attempted a complete separation of the physiological and pathological and have tended to reject all observations which relate to tissues which are in any way pathological. In many instances, however, the border line between these two concepts is so diffuse that division is impossible. Thus, although age changes in bone can result in frank osteoporosis, a certain proportion of subjects present with a degree of bone damage which is well outside the statistically permissible limits (p. 52). Discussion of these has been included in this volume, for the simple reason, that by their very existence they provide information which is of use in an assessment of the "physiological" changes. Similarly, a study of age changes in the plasma elastase levels in cases of pseudoxanthoma elasticum, (p. 157) has been included in the section dealing with connective tissue degradation, since the observations made on these plasmas have proved of interest in an assessment of age changes in the normal population.

One of the most difficult areas for gerontologists to work in has been that of the cardiovascular system, since here the separation of age and pathology has proved particularly intractable. The fundamental changes in the structure and function of the vessel walls which are associated with the development of atherosclerotic lesions may, however, be justifiably classified as ageing phenomena, since they satisfy the criteria for true ageing put forward by Strehler, 1962, (p. 2).

Vascular diseases

The effect of hypertension on vascular proteins

Berry (1973) has shown that the elastin content of vascular tissue increases considerably at birth when there are marked changes in the tension in the vessel wall. Wolinsky (1970) has demonstrated that such changes both in elastin and collagen content are not restricted to the neonatal period, but under proper stimulation can continue throughout life, especially under conditions in which the animal or human subject becomes hypertensive, for either experimental or pathological reasons. The absolute levels of elastin and collagen are the important factors here, for, as Sandberg (1975) points out, measurement of the ratios of one to the other cannot provide unequivocal information regarding the changes in structure which occur.

Atherosclerosis and vascular proteins

The distensibility of the aortas of cholesterol-fed animals has been shown to increase dramatically (Burton, 1954; Newman et al., 1971). The latter group has demonstrated that there is a direct correlation between the atherogenic index of the blood vessels and their distensibility, possibly due to a weakening of the mass of elastin and collagen which lies between pairs of medial lamellae.

It has long been appreciated that one of the criteria of the development of aortic lesions following the administration of cholesterol in the diet is the fragmentation and re-synthesis of the elastin of the internal elastic lamina. Part of this phenomenon is degradative, but the appearance of new elastic fibres, and the infiltration of glycoproteins may be ascribed to a reparative process. Saxl and Hall (1967) have demonstrated the conversion of a lipid-poor form of elastic tissue in the aortas of young chickens into a lipid-rich complex following the administration of cholesterol. The elastic tissue becomes degraded, and can be located in the vessel wall in the form of globules. On the approach of cholesterol, following its penetration into the vascular tissue, the globules uncoil and align themselves parallel to the lipid-cholesterol mycelles which can be identified by their osmophilic properties in the electron microscope (Fig. 71). The two then combine with the production of a lipoprotein complex which is not as osmophilic as the original lipid mycelle. Kramsch et al. (1974) injected tritiated cholesterol into moribund subjects. and observed the location of the steroid to be in close association with re-duplicated or fragmented elastic membranes. No association between cholesterol and intact elastin was observed. They also noticed that the association of cholesterol and elastin as in the atherosclerotic plaque protected 25% of

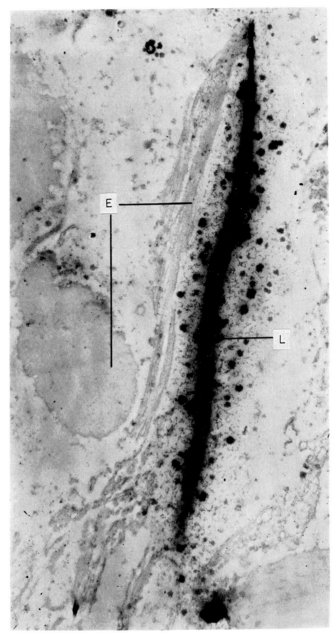

FIG. 71. The appearance of elastin protein-lipid complexes in the aortic tissue of the chick following the administration of a cholesterol-rich diet for a period of 6 months. E, elastin; L, lipid. (×19 000)

the elastin from digestion by elastase. The 75% of the plaque elastin, which could be dissolved by the enzyme, separated into two fractions on Sephadex G200, whereas elastolysates of normal elastin consisted of a single fraction which was identical with one of the plaque fractions. The other fraction which was unique to plaque elastin could be shown to be a lipopolypeptide by virtue of its stainability with both Amidoschwarz and oil red O, and proved to contain about 44% of a lipid, which was mainly cholesterol ester. Band *et al.* (1973) observed a 50% increase in rigidity (expressed in terms of Young's Modulus) in segments of aortas from rabbits and rats rendered atherosclerotic by cholesterol-rich diets, thus demonstrating that even the slight changes in structure associated with the association of elastin and cholesterol are sufficient to alter the physical properties of the wall to a considerable extent.

Elastase and atherosclerosis

The involvement of elastase in the development of atherosclerotic lesions or in its prevention, as opposed to its role in the ageing of the connective tissues of the artery walls, has been the subject of a number of research projects over the past 20 years. The whole question, however, has been confused by the inclusion of extraneous enzyme systems in many of the elastase preparations which have been studied. Hall (1961a) was the first to attempt to disentangle the effects of the proteolytic component of the elastase complex, elasto-proteinase, from the mucolytic and lipolytic enzymes which are produced in association with it in the pancreas, and which have contaminated many of the earlier crude preparations of the proteolytic enzyme. These non-elastolytic enzymes are dealt with in detail in the section on lipolytic systems on p. 163. Their effective separation from elastase itself has cleared up much of the early confusion, in which it was suggested that "elastase" had lipolytic, and anti-cholesterolaemic activity (cf. p. 162).

Loeven (1965a) confirmed Hall's (1953, 1958, 1961b) division of the elastase complex into a variety of components and provided evidence for the presence in the pancreas of two forms of a proteolytic enzyme to both of which the name elastase could be given. These have more recently (Hall, 1971; Tesal, 1971; Tesal and Hall, 1972; Hall and Tesal, 1976) been identified as a calcium-poor (E) and a calcium-rich (ECa) form of the enzyme (p. 133), and the possibility of a direct involvement of these enzymes in arterial wall degeneration during the development of age-related atherosclerosis has been studied.

Balo and Banga (1955) determined the amounts of elastase present in the pancreases of subjects with arterial lesions of varying degrees of severity, and used this rather than age as their yard stick. They observed a marked reduction in the amount of enzyme in the pancreases of subjects with severe atherosclerosis. It may be assumed that the majority of these would have been in older age groups, and hence the reduction in elastase content could be equally attributable to age and atherosclerosis. Loeven (1970) on the other hand, compared the amounts of both E and ECa forms of elastase in the pancreases of subjects with a "normal" degree of atherosclerosis and with severe involvement, in four age groups from 50 to 90 years of age, thus permitting the relative effects of age and atherosclerosis to be differentiated. As might be expected the severity of atherosclerosis was greatest in males and in older age groups. The mean value for the amount of the calcium-poor form of the enzyme in the normal male pancreas fell from 0.75 units/g in the 50–60-year old group to 0.4 units/g at age 80–90, whereas the level in the pancreases of males with severe atherosclerosis was lower throughout life (c. 0.25 units/g), and only fell slightly (to 0.2 units/g) in the oldest group. The level of ECa shows similar variations with age in the case of the "normal" subjects, and the universally low value which is typical of those with severe atherosclerosis throughout life. In general this form of enzyme is present at about five times higher concentration than the E form, and this is approximately true at all ages.

Elastase levels in female pancreases are similarly low in those subjects with severe atherosclerosis at all ages from 50 to 90, the reduction in elastase content which occurs in the pancreases of all "normal" females (cf. p. 156) in the peri-menopausal decade being completely eliminated.

These observations are of considerable importance in view of the recent findings (Chatterjee, 1975) that plasma levels of elastase are significantly higher than normal in the case of subjects with some form of cardiac or cerebral involvement at all ages above 60.

Deposition of lipid in arterial connective tissues

A considerable amount of lipid is stored in the endothelial cells of the artery wall, but also extracellularly between the elastic lamellae and the collagen fibres. Even in infant tissues fatty streaks have been observed (Lev and Sullivan, 1951; Holman, 1961), but there is still considerable controversy as to whether these deposits represent the beginning of changes which can be associated directly with the ageing process, are the first stage in the development of atherosclerotic lesion or are in fact not directly associated with either of these conditions.

The increasing amount of lipid which is present in human arterial tissues at all ages above infancy does not represent an enhancement of all classes of lipid across the board. The level of cholesterol ester, initially one of the least important contributors to the overall lipid spectrum, increases rapidly, until in aged tissues it represents the major lipid component. The nature of the fatty acid which esterifies the cholesterol does not remain constant throughout life, the linoleic acid component of the cholesterol ester fraction of the aorta as a whole, increasing more rapidly than other esterifying fatty acids (Smith,

1965). The fatty streaks, however, which appear early in the development of arterial lipoidosis are rich in oleic acid and its metabolic product, eicosotrienoic acid. Slater (1966) and Smith *et al.* (1967) have demonstrated that there is a marked difference between the perifibrous lipid and this intracellular fraction, in that the former appears from its fatty acid composition to be derived from the Sf O-12 lipoproteins of the plasma, whereas the latter, from its oleic acid-rich nature, may be assumed to be synthesised *in situ* from circulating acetate.

The manner in which the perifibrous lipid becomes bound to the elastin, collagen or pseudoelastin in the vessel wall is by no means clear, nor has it yet been proved unequivocally how lipid from the circulation penetrates the vessel wall. It may be that it penetrates from the lumen of the vessel by diffusion through intercellular junctions or defects in the endothelial layer (Bondjers, 1972) or by pincnocytosis (Stein and Stein, 1973) or from the *vasa vasorum* which serves the outer layers of the wall (Caro, 1973). Once the lipid has penetrated into the wall, it may be retained within the network of fibres and lamellae, either by direct interaction with the elastin molecules (Saxl and Hall, 1967) or with glycosaminoglycans (Iverius, 1973). The identity of at least part of the elastic fibre as a lipoprotein has been confirmed by studies of the interaction of elastolipoproteinase, a member of the elastase complex, as isolated in crude form from the pancreas, on intact elastic tissue (Saxl, 1957a). Elastase alone is not adequate for the optimal dissolution of elastic tissue present in unfixed frozen sections of aorta. Saxl showed, and Loeven confirmed (1965b) that a preparation containing both elastolipoproteinase and elastomucase had to be added to the proteolytic enzyme, if the untreated tissue were to dissolve at a rapid rate, or the tissue had to be pretreated with the non-proteolytic preparation. Saxl (1957b) also showed that the relative amounts of the two enzymes required for an optimal rate of dissolution differed for tissues of differing age. Tissue from a 12-year old child was essentially resistant to attack by elastase alone, for periods up to 17 h, and the addition of lipolytic and mucolytic enzymes was without effect. Tissue from a 36-year old subject is also resistant to rapid dissolution by elastase alone, but this situation can be altered if the tissue is pretreated with the elastomucase/elastolipoproteinase mixture. Sixty-four-year old tissue on the other hand can be easily degraded by elastase alone in $6\frac{1}{2}$ h. Saxl and Hall (1967) were of the opinion that the major part of this differential age effect was due to the mucolytic activity of the elastomucase, but it has since become apparent (Loeven, 1969) that the preparation they were using contained both mucolytic and lipolytic elements, and hence, although part of the stability of the tissue in the young and middle-aged subjects might be due to the interaction of elastin protein and a glycosaminoglycan entity, it is also possible that the addition of lipid might be of importance in this respect.

Miller (1971) has identified an enzyme system in the pancreas which can be isolated together with elastase in crude preparations which has many of the properties of a lipoprotein lipase, and Loeven (1963) has demonstrated a similar enzyme in plasma and in the arterial wall (Loeven, 1969). All these preparations combine their activity with that of elastase itself to produce a synergistically greater response in the dissolution of elastin with the liberation into the medium of free fatty acids in addition to protein degradation products.

Changes in glycosaminoglycan content of atheromatous vessel walls

Studies on the distribution of glycosaminoglycans in human arterial tissue has given very inconsistent results. Hyaluronic acid has invariably been shown to be reduced in amount in advanced age, but dermatan sulphate, heparan sulphate and chondroitin sulphate have often been shown to increase in amounts, (Kaplan and Meyer, 1960; Manley *et al.*, 1969; Dalferes *et al.*, 1971). However, measurement of the incorporation of ^{35}S-sulphate into the sulphated glycosaminoglycans as a whole (Hauss, *et al.* 1968; Sanwald *et al.*, 1971), has demonstrated that an increased synthesis of these compounds is an immediate accompaniment of the onset of arteriosclerosis, whereas the metabolic activity of these systems, which bring about such syntheses appears to be reduced in age. Buddecke *et al.* (1973) have studied the incorporation of ^{35}S in bovine aorta, in order to eliminate the atherosclerotic element. Between birth and $12\frac{1}{2}$ years of age, there were no significant differences in the overall proportions of chrondroitin sulphate, which accounted for 50% of the total glycosaminoglycan, dermatan sulphate which amounted to 25% and heparan sulphate and hyaluronic acid, which were respectively 10% and 15% of the total. The total amount of glycosaminoglycan rose dramatically over the first three years of life from 1.8 to 3.4 mg/g wet tissue and then fell progressively over the next seven years to a value of 2.3 mg/g.

The incorporation of ^{35}S-sulphate into the three sulphated glycosaminoglycans expressed as cpm/mg of each, fell off exponentially with age, but it can be calculated from the figures presented by Buddecke *et al.* (1973) that the reduction in sulphate incorporation as calculated from the changing proportion of the glycosaminoglycan in the tissue is more nearly linear. If, however, the rate of reduction in incorporation is plotted against the tissue DNA level, it can be seen that each cell retains its activity almost unabated throughout life, the incorporation of ^{35}S-sulphate in cpm/μ mol DNA remaining within 8% of its mean value until the eighth year of life, and then only dropping by a further 11% in later years.

Lindner and Johannes (1973) observed similar rates of fall of ^{35}S-sulphate incorporation during the maturation and ageing of human and rat aortas. In the latter tissue, however, they reported an almost linear fall in the rate of incorporation of ^{35}S per unit DNA as compared with the similar relationship for rat dermis in which the cellular activity was maintained as in bovine aorta.

References

Abrahams, M. (1967). 7th Int. Conf. of Med. and Biol. Engineering, p. 509. Stockholm, Almqvist and Wiksell.

Adams, E. (1970). *Internat. Revs. Connective Tissue Res.* **5**, 1.

Aer, J. and Kivirikko, K. I. (1969). *Hoppe-Seylers Z. Physiol. Chem.* **350**, 87.

Alexander, R. McN. (1962). *J. Exp. Biol.* **39**, 373.

Allalauf, D. A. and Ber, A. (1961). *Endocrinology*, **69**, 210.

Amati, A. and Castelli, B. (1961). *Ital. J. Biochem.* **10**, 292.

Aminoff, D. (1961). *Biochem. J.* **81**, 384.

Anderson, J. A. and Jackson, D. S. (1972). *Biochem. J.* **127**, 179.

Anderson, S. O. (1964). *Biochem. Biophys. Acta.* **93**, 213.

Anderson, S. O. (1966). *Acta Physiol. Scand.* **66**, Suppl. 263.

Andrew, W. (1938). *Z. Zellforsch. Mikrosk. Anat.* **28**, 294.

Anon. (1962). *Chem. Eng. News*, **40**, Feb. 12, p. 138; Feb. 19, p. 104.

Armstrong, J. R. (1965). "Lumbar Disc Lesions", 3rd ed. Edinburgh, Churchill, Livingstone.

Asboe-Hansen, G. (1966). "Hormones and Connective Tissues". Copenhagen, Munksgaard.

Astbury, W. T. (1938). *Trans. Faraday Soc.* **34**, 377.

Astbury, W. T. and Bell, F. O. (1940). *Nature, London*, **145**, 421.

Avioli, L. V., McDonald, J. E., Henneman, P. H. and Lee, S. W. (1966). *J. Clin. Invest.* **45**, 1093.

Ayer, J. P. (1964). *Int. Revs. Connective Tissue Res.* **2**, 33.

Ayer, J. P., Hass, G. M. and Philpott, D. F. (1958). *Arch. Path.* **63**, 519.

Bagdy, D., Tolnay, P., Borsy, J. and Kovacs, K. (1960). *Magyar Tudomanyos Akad. Biol. es Orvosi Tudomanyok Osztalynak Köslemenyei*, **11**, 277.

Bailey, A. J. (1967). *Biochem. J.* **105**, 34.

Bailey, A. J. (1969). *Gerontologia*, **15**, 65.

Bailey, A. J. and Peach, C. M. (1968). *Biochem. Biophys. Res. Commun.* **33**, 812.

Bailey, A. J. and Shimokomaki, M. (1971). *F.E.B.S. Letters*, **16**, 86.

Bailey, A. J. and Robins, S. P. (1972). *F.E.B.S. Letters*, **21**, 330.

Bailey, A. J. and Robins, S. P. (1973). *In* "Frontiers of Matrix Biology. 1. Ageing of Connective Tissue. Skin" (Eds Robert, L. and Robert, B.), p. 130. Basel, Karger.

Baker, S. P., Gaffney, G. W. and Shock, N. W. (1959). *J. Gerontol.* **24**, 37.

Bakerman, S. (1962). *Nature, London*, **196**, 375.

Bakerman, S. (1964). *Biochem. Biophys. Acta*, **90**, 621.

Balazs, E. A. (1968). *Ber. 68th Zusammenkunft Deut. Ophthalm. Ges.* p. 536.

Balo, J. and Banga, I. (1949). *Schweiz Z. Pathol. u. Bakteriol.* **12**, 350.

Balo, J. and Banga, I. (1950). *Biochem. J.* **46**, 384.

Balo, J. and Banga, I. (1955). *Proc. 3rd Internat. Congr. Biochem.* **14**, 3, 120.

Balo, J., Banga, I. and Szabo, D. (1956). *Magy. Tud. Akad. Biol. Orv. Oszt. Közl.* **7**, 385.

Band, W., Goodhard, W. J. and Knoop, A. A. (1973). *Atherosclerosis*, **18**, 163.

Baldauf, L.K. (1906) *J. Med. Res.* **15**, 355.

Banga, I. (1953). *Nature, London*, **172**, 1099.

Banga, I. (1966). "Structure and Function of Elastin and Collagen". Budapest, Akademiai Kaido.

Banga, I. (1969). *Int. Symp. Biochem. Vascular Wall. Fribourg*, 1968 II 18.

Banga, I. and Ardelt, W. (1967). *Biochim. Biophys. Acta*, **146**, 284.

Banga, I. and Balo, J. (1956). *Nature, London*, **178**, 310.

Banga, I., Balo, J. and Szabo, D. (1956). *J. Gerontol.* **11**, 242.

Barnett, C. H., Davies, D. V. and MacConaill, M. A. (1961). "Synovial Joints – Their Structure and Mechanics". New York, Longmans Green.

Barrett, A. J. and Dingle, J. T. (1971). "Tissue Proteinases". Amsterdam, North Holland Publishing Co.

Barrows, C. H. (1956). *Fed. Proc.* **15**, 954.

Bartelheimer, H., Kulpe, W. and Somerkamp, H. (1958). *Klin. Woechenschr.* **36**, 780.

Becker, B. and Collier, E. (1965). *Invest. Ophthalmol.* **4**, 117.

Bencosme, S. A. and Craston, D. F. (1958). *Lab. Invest.* **7**, 201.

Berg, B. N. (1956). *J. Gerontol.* **11**, 134.

Berry, C. L. (1973). *Ann. Roy. Coll. Surg. Engl.* **53**, 246.

Berry, C. L. and Looker, J. (1973). *J. Anat.* **114**, 83.

Berry, C. L., Looker, T. and Germain, J. (1972). *J. Anat.* **113**, 1.

Bertolini, A. M. (1962). *Gerontologia*, **6**, 175.

Bjorksten, J. (1958). *J. Amer. Geriatrics Soc.* **6**, 740.

Bjorksten, J. (1968). *J. Amer. Geriatrics Soc.* **16**, 408.

Blakey, P. R., Happey, F., Naylor, A. and Turner, R. L. (1962). *Nature, London*, **194**, 73.

Blumenthal, H. T., Lansing, A. I. and Gray, S. H. (1950). *Amer. J. Path.* **26**, 989.

Blumgart, H. L., Gilligan, D. R. and Schlesinger, M. J. (1940). *Trans. Ass. Amer. Phys.* **55**, 313.

Boisson, H., Pieraggi, M. T., Julian, M. and Blazy, L. D. (1973). *In* "Frontiers of Matrix Biology, 1. Ageing of Connective Tissue. Skin" (Eds Robert, L. and Robert, B.), p. 190. Basel, Karger.

Bolick, L. I. and Blankenhorn, D. H. (1961). *Am. J. Path.* **39**, 511.

Bonjers, G. (1972). Thesis, University of Gothenburg, quoted by Iveruis (1973).

Bornstein, P. (1972). *In* "The Comparative Molecular Biology of Extra-cellular Matrices" (Ed. Slavkin, H. C.), p. 309. New York, Academic Press.

Bornstein, P., Ehrlich, H. P. and Wyke, A. W. (1972). *Science*, **175**, 544.

Bornstein, P. and Piez, K. A. (1964). *J. Clin. Invest.* **43**, 1813.

Bornstein, P. and Piez, K. A. (1966). *Biochemistry*, **5**, 3460.

Bornstein, P., Martin, G. R. and Piez, K. A. (1964). *Science*, **144**, 1220.

Bourne, G. H. (1951). "Cytology and Cell Physiology", 2nd ed. Oxford, Clarendon Press.

Bourne, G. H. (1957). *Nature, London*, **179**, 472.

Bowen, T.J. (1953). *Biochem. J.* **55**, 766.

Branwell, A. W. (1963). *Internat. Revs. Connective Tissue Res.* **1**, 1.

Braun-Falco, O. (1956). *Dermat. Wochenschr.* **134**, 1022.

Braun-Falco, O. and Salfeld, K. (1957a). *Dermat. Wochenschr.* **135**, 370.

Braun-Falco, O. and Salfeld, K. (1957b). *Dermat. Wochenschr.* **135**, 374.

Brocas, J. and Verzar, F. (1961). *Gerontologia*, **5**, 228.

Brown, P. C., Consden, R. and Glynn, L. E. (1958). *Ann. Rheumatol. Dis.* **17**, 196.

Brown-Séquard, C. E. (1889). *C.R. Soc. Biol.* **41**, 415.

Brunet, P. C. J. and Kent, P. W. (1955). *Proc. Roy. Soc. B.* **144**, 259.

Bruns, R. R. and Gross, J. (1973). *Biochem.* **12**, 808.

Buddecke, E. (1958). *Hoppe-Seylers Z. Physiol. Chem.* **310**, 182.

Buddecke, E. and Kresse, H. (1974). *In* "Connective Tissues – Biochemistry and Pathophysiology" (Eds Fricke, R. and Hartmann, F.), p. 131. Berlin, Springer Verlag.

Buddecke, E., Kroz, W. and Tittor, W. (1967). *Hoppe-Seylers Z. Physiol. Chem.* **348**, 651.

Buddecke, E., Segeth, G. and Kresse, H. (1973a). *In* "Connective Tissue and Ageing" (Ed. Vogel, H. G.), p. 62. Amsterdam, Excerpta Medica.

Buddecke, E., Wellauer, P. and Wyler, T. (1973b). *In* "Connective Tissue and Ageing" (Ed. Vogel, H. G.), p. 140. Amsterdam, Excerpta Medica.

Buddecke, E. and Siegoleits, M. (1964). *Hoppe-Seylers Z. Physiol. Chem.* **337**, 105.

Bullough, W. S. (1967). "Evolution and Differentiation". New York, Academic Press.

Bullough, W. S. (1973). *In* "Hormonal Control of Growth and Differentiation" (Eds Le Bue, J. and Gordon, A. S.), Vol. 2, p. 3. New York, Academic Press.

Bullough, W. S. and Laurence, E. B. (1960a). *Proc. Roy. Soc. B.* **151**, 517.

Bullough, W. S. and Laurence, E. B. (1960b). *Exptl. Cell. Res.* **21**, 394.

Bullough, W. S. and Laurence, E. B. (1971). Unpublished, quoted in Bullough 1973.

Bullough, W. S., Hewett, C. L. and Laurence, E. B. (1964). *Exptl. Cell. Res.* **36**, 192.

Buck, R. C. (1951). *Arch. Pathol.* **51, 319.**

Buck, R. C. (1954). *AMA Arch. Pathol.* **58**, 576.

Buonocore, G. (1958). *Ann. della Spec. Agraria, Roma,* **12**, 681.

Burrows, F. G. O. (1965). *Brit. J. Radiol.* **38**, 309.

Burton, A. C. (1954). *Physiol. Rev.* **34**, 619.

Burton, A. C. (1967). *Gastroenterol.* **52**, 363.

Burton, D., Hall, D. A., Keech, M. K., Reed, R., Saxl, H., Tunbridge, R. E. and Wood, M. J. (1955). *Nature, London,* **176**, 966.

Butturini, U., Giro, C. and Langer, M. (1959a). *Boll. Soc. Ital. Biol. Sper.* **35**, 33.

Butturini, U., Langer, M. and Giro, C. (1959b). *Boll. Soc. Ital. Biol. Sper.* **35**, 30.

Butturini, U., Pretolani, E. and Gnudi, A. (1959c). *Boll. Soc. Ital. Biol. Sper.* **35**, 27.

Cacciola, E., Cristaldi, R. and Guistolisi, R. (1963). *Arch. Ricambio,* **27**, 681.

Cadavid, N. G., Denduchis, B. and Mancini, R. E. (1963). *Lab. Invest.* **12**, 598.

Campagnari, F. and Greggia, G. (1959). *Minerva. Med., Torino,* **50**, 2899.

Carlborg, U. (1944). *Acta. Med. Scand. Suppl.* **151**, 205.

Caro, C. G. (1973). *In* "Atherogenesis: Initiating factors", *Ciba Foundation Symposium,* **12**, 127, Amsterdam, Elsevier.

Carr, I. (1973). "The Macrophage". London, Academic Press.

Carter, A. E. (1956). *Science,* **123**, 669.

Chapelle, C. de la and Cohn, A. (1931). *Am. J. Anat.* **49**, 241.

Chapman, J. A. (1966. *In* "Principles of Biomolecular Organization" (Eds Wolstenholme, J. E. W. and O'Connor, M.), p. 129. London, Churchill.

Chapman, J. A. (1974). *Connective Tissue Res.* **2**, 137.

Chatterjee, J. (1975). *Age and Ageing,* **4**, 129.

Chvapil, M. (1959). *Cesk. Fysiol.* **8**, 81.

Chvapil, M. and Hurych, J. (1968). *Int. Revs. Connective Tissue Res.* **4**, 68.

Chvapil, M. and Jensovsky, L. (1963). *Gerontologia,* **7**, 18.

Cifonelli, J. A., Ludowieg, J. and Dorfman, A. (1958). *J. Biol. Chem.* **233**, 541.

Citi, S., Leone, O., Salvini, L., Grandonico, F. and Viola, S. (1960). *Giorn. Gerontol.* **8,** 576, 581.

Clark, C. C. (1976). *In* "Methodology of Connective Tissue Research" (Ed. Hall, D. A.), p. 205. Oxford, Joynson-Bruvvers.

Clausen, B. (1962). *Lab. Invest.* **11,** 1340.

Cleary, E. G. and McCloskey, D. I. (1962). *Aust. J. Sci.* **25,** 110.

Cleary, E. G., Sandberg, L. B. and Jackson, D. S. (1966). *J. Cell. Biol.* **33,** 469.

Cliff, W. J. (1971). *Exptl. and Mol. Pathol.* **43,** 945.

Cohen, H., Megel, H. and Kleinberg, W. (1958). *Proc. Soc. Exptl. Biol. Med.* **97,** 8.

Comfort, A. (1956). "Ageing, the Biology of Senescence". London, Routledge, and Kegan Paul.

Cooper, D. R. and Davidson, R. J. (1965). *Biochem. J.* **97,** 139.

Cotton, R. and Wartman, W. B. (1961). *Arch. Path. Chicago,* **71,** 3.

Cowan, P. M., North, A. C. T. and Randall, J. T. (1955). *Symp. Exptl. Biol.* **9,** 115.

Cox, H. T. (1941). *Brit. J. Surg.* **29,** 234.

Cox, R. C. and Little, K. (1961). *Proc. Roy. Soc. B,* **155,** 232.

Craciun, E. C. (1973). *Scand. J. Clin. Lab. Invest.* Suppl. **141,** 41.

Craik, J. E. and McNeil, I. R. R. (1966). *Nature, London,* **209,** 931.

Crick, F. H. C. (1954). *J. Chem. Phys.* **22,** 347.

Cronkite, A. E. (1936). *Anat. Rec.* **64,** 173.

Curtis, H. J., Leith, J. and Tilley, J. (1966). *J. Geront.* **21,** 365.

Czerkawski, J. W. (1962). *Nature, London,* **194,** 869.

Dabbous, M. K. (1966). *J. Biol. Chem.* **241,** 5307.

Dagliotti, G. C. (1931). *Z. Anat. und Entwickl. Gesch.* **96,** 680.

Dalfres, E. R., Ruiz, H., Kumer, V., Radhakrisnamurthy, B. and Berenson, G. S. (1971). *Artherosclerosis,* **13,** 121.

Daly, C. H. (1969). Cited by Millington *et al.* in Proc. 8th Internat. Conf. on Mechanical and Biological Engineering, p. 18. Tokyo, 1971.

Danielli, J. F. (1956). *Experientia, Suppl.* **4,** 55.

Davidson, E. A. and Woodhall, B. (1959). *J. Biol. Chem.* **234,** 2951.

Davis, N. R. and Bailey, A. J. (1971). *Biochem. Biophys. Res. Commun.* **45,** 1416.

Dawber, R. and Shuster, S. (1971). *Brit. J. Dermatol.* **84,** 130.

Dehm, P., Jimenez, S. A., Olsen, B. R. and Prockop, P. J. (1972). *Proc. Nat. Acad. Sci. U.S.* **69,** 60.

Dent, C. E. and Watson, L. (1966). "Osteoporosis", *Postgrad. Med. J. Suppl.* 583.

Dequeker, J., Remans, J., Fransses, R. and Waes, J. (1971). *Calc. Tiss. Res.* **7,** 23

Dick, J. C. (1947). *J. Anat.* **81,** 201.

Dick, J. C. (1951). *J. Physiol., Lond.* **112,** 102.

Dische, Z. and Zelmenis, G. (1955). *A.M.A. Arch. Ophthalmol.* **54,** 528.

Doljanski, L. and Romlet, F. C. (1933). *Arch. Pathol. Anat. u. Physiol. Virchow,* **291,** 260.

Dorfman, A. (1970). *In* "Chemistry and Molecular Biology of the Intercellular Matrix", p. 1421, (Ed. Balazs, E. A.). Vol. 3 New York, Academic Press.

Dowson, D., Longfield, M. D., Walker, P. S. and Wright, V. (1968). *Proc. Inst. Mech. Eng.* **182N,** 68.

Dupuytren, G. (1834). "Traite des Blessures, par Armes de Guerre", Vol. 1, p. 66. Paris, Baillière.

Ebel, A., Mack, G. and Fontaine, J. L. (1970). *Path. Biol., Paris,* **18,** 59, 69.

Eddy, D. D. and Farber, E. M. (1962). *Arch. Dermatol.* **86,** 729.

Ehrenberg, R., Winnecken, H. G. and Biebricher, H. (1954). *Z. Naturforsch.* **96,** 492.

Ehrich, W., Chappelle, C. de la and Cohn, A. (1931). *Amer. J. Path.* **33,** 525.

Eisen, A. Z. (1969). *J. Invest. Dermatol.* **52,** 442.

Eisen, A. Z., Jeffrey, J. J. and Gross, J. (1968). *Biochim. Biophys. Acta.* **151,** 637.

Eisenthal, R. and Cornish-Bowden, A. (1974). *Biochem. J.* **139,** 715.

Ejiri, I. (1936). *Jap. J. Dermatol. Urol.* **40,** 46, 173, 216.

Ejiri, I. (1937). *Jap. J. Dermatol. Urol.* **41,** 8, 64, 95.

Elden, H. R. (1965). *Adv. Biol. Skin.* **6,** 229.

Elden, H. R. (1966). *In* "Perspectives in Experimental Gerontology" (Ed. Shock, N. W.), p. 83. Springfield, C. C. Thomas.

Elden, H. R. (1970). *In* "Advances in Biology of Skin. The Dermis", Vol. X, p. 392. New York, Wiley-Interscience.

Elden, H. R. and Boucek, R. J. (1962). *In* "Biological Aspects of Aging" (Ed. Shock, N. W.). New York, Columbia University Press.

Elliot, D. H. (1965). *Biol. Revs.* **40,** 392.

Elliott, D. H. (1967). *Ann. Phys. Med.* **9,** 1.

Evans, H. M. and Scott, K. J. (1921). *Carnegie Inst. Contrib. Embryology*, **10,** 1.

Evanson, J. M. (1976). *In* "The Chemistry and Molecular Biology of the Intercellular Matrix" (Ed. Balazs, E. A.), p. 1637. New York, Academic Press.

Evanson, J. (1975). *In* "Methodology of Connective Tissue Research" (Ed. Hall, D. A.), p. 175. Oxford, Joynson-Bruvvers.

Evanson, J. M., Jeffrey, J. J. and Krane, S. M. (1967). *Science*, **158,** 499.

Evanson, J. M., Minkin, C. and Reynolds, J. (1970). *J. Bone Jt. Surg.* **52B,** 182.

Everitt, A. V. (1971). *Gerontologia*, **17,** 98.

Everitt, A. V. and Olsen, G. G. (1965). *Nature, London*, **206,** 307.

Evald, A. (1890). *Z. Biol.* **26,** 1.

Exton-Smith, A. N. (1973). *In* "Textbook of Geriatric Medicine and Gerontology" (Ed. Brocklehurst, J. C.), p. 476. Edinburgh, Churchill, Livingstone.

Feitelberg, S. and Kaunitz, P. E. (1949). *Biochim. Biophys. Acta.* **3,** 155.

Fels, I. G. (1966). *J. Amer. Leather Chem. Ass.* **61,** 351.

Fessler, J. H. and Bailey, A. J. (1965). *Fed. Proc.* **25,** 1022.

Findlay, G. H. (1954). *Brit. J. Dermatol.* **66,** 16.

Fine, B. S. and Tousimis, A. J. (1961). *Arch. Ophthalmol.* **65,** 95

Finean, J. B. (1967). "Biological Structure". New York, Academic Press.

Fitzpatrick, M. J. and Hospelhorn, V. D. (1960). *J. Lab. Clin. Med.* **56,** 812.

Flately, F. J., Atwell, M. E. and McEvoy, R. K. (1963). *Arch. Intern. Med.* **112,** 352.

Fleischmajer, R., Perlish, J. S. and Bashey, R. I. (1973). *In* "Frontiers of Matrix Biology. 1. Ageing of Connective Tissue. Skin" (Eds Robert, L. and Robert, B.), p. 90. Basel, Karger.

Foster, J. A., Gray, W. R. and Franzblau, C. (1973). *Biochem. Biophys. Acta.* **303,** 363.

Foster, J. A., Rubin L., Kagar, H. M. and Franzblau, C. (1974). *J. Biol. Chem.* **249,** 6191.

Francis, G., John, R. and Thomas, J. (1973). *Biochem. J.* **136,** 45.

Franks, L. M., Wilson, P. D. and Whelan, R. D. (1974). *Gerontologia*, **20,** 21.

Fransson, L. A. (1970). *In* "Chemistry and Molecular Biology of the Intercellular Matrix" (Ed. Balazs, E. A.), Vol. 2, p. 823. New York, Academic Press.

Fransson, L. A. and Rodén, L. (1967). *J. Biol. Chem.* **242,** 4161, 4170.

Franzblau, C. (1971). *In* "Comprehensive Biochemistry" (Eds Florkin, M. and Stotz, E. H.), Vol. 26, p. 659. New York, Elsevier.

Franzblau, C., Sinex, F. M., Faris, B. and Lampidis, R. (1965). *Biochim. Biophys. Res. Commun.* **21**, 575.

Freeman, E. (1973). *In* "Textbook of Geriatric Medicine and Gerontology" (Ed. Brocklehurst, J. C.), p. 405. Edinburgh, Churchill, Livingstone.

Frost, H. M. and Villaneuva, A. R. (1960). *Stain. Technol.* **35**, 179.

Fujimori, E. (1966). *Biochemistry*, **5**, 1034.

Fullmer, H. M. and Lazarus, G. S. (1967). *Nature, London*, **209**, 728.

Fullmer, H. M. and Lillie, R. D. (1957). *J. Histochem. Cytochem.* **4**, 64.

Fung, Y. C. B. (1967). *Amer. J. Physiol.* **213**, 1532.

Galante, J. O. (1967). *Acta Orthopt. Scand.* Suppl. 100.

Gallop, P. M., Seifter, S. and Meilman, E. (1959). *Nature, London*, **183**, 1659.

Gazert, P. (1898). *Deutsch. Arch. Klin. Med.* **62**, 390.

Geokas, M. C., Wilding, P., Rinderknecht, H. and Haverback, B. J. (1968). *Clin. Biochem.* **1**, 251.

Gerber, G. E. and Anwar, R. A. (1974). *J. Biol. Chem.* **249**, 5200.

Ghiringhelli, E. M., Mira, E. and Gerzell, G. (1963). *Giron. Geront.* **11**, 1097.

Gilfillan, R. F., Sbarra, A. J. and Bardawil, W. A. (1960). *Fed. Proc.* **19**, 144.

Gilfillan, R. F., Sbarra, A. J. and Bardawil, W. A. (1961). *Fed. Proc.* **20**, 161.

Gillman, T., Penn, J., Bronks, D. and Roux, M. (1955a). *Arch. Pathol.* **59**, 733.

Gillman, T., Penn, J., Bronks, D. and Roux, M. (1955b). *Brit. J. Cancer.* **9**, 272.

Glaser, A. A., Maragoni, R. D., Must, J. S., Beckwith, T. G., Brody, G. S., Walker, G. R. and White, W. L. (1965). *Med. Electron. Biol. Engineer*, **3**, 411.

Good, M. (1958). *Zeit. Ges. Inn. Med.* **13**, 28.

Gore, L. and Larkey, B. J. (1960). *J. Lab. Clin. Med.* **56**, 839.

Gould, B. S. (1968). *In* "Treatise on Collagen" (Ed. Gould, B. S.), Vol. 2A, p. 139. London, Academic Press.

Gould, B. S. (1968). *Int. Revs. Connective Tissue Res.* **4**, 35.

Graham, G. N. (1958). Ph.D. Thesis, University of Leeds.

Grahame, R. and Holt, P. J. L. (1969). *Gerontologia*, **15**, 121.

Grant, N. H. and Alburn, H. E. (1965). *Biochemistry*, **4**, 127.

Grant, N. H. and Robbins, K. C. (1955). *Proc. Soc. Exptl. Biol. Med.* **90**, 264.

Grant, R. A. (1966). *Brit. J. Exptl. Pathol.* **47**, 163.

Greiling, H. and Baumann, G. (1973). *In* "Connective Tissue and Ageing" (Ed. Vogel, H.), p. 160. Amsterdam, Excerpta Medica.

Grillo, H. C. and Gross, J. (1967). *Develop. Biol.* **15**, 300.

Gross, J. (1963). *Biochim. Biophys. Acta.* **71**, 250.

Gustavson, K. H. (1956). "The Chemistry and Reactivity of Collagen". New York, Academic Press.

Hahn, H. P. von (1964). *Gerontologia*, **10**, 107, 174.

Hahn, H. P. von (1971). *In* "Molekulare und Zellulare Aspekte des Alterns" (Eds Platt, D. and Lasch, H. G.), p. 125. Stuttgart, Schaltauer.

Hall, D. A. (1951). *Nature, London*, **168**, 513.

Hall, D. A. (1953). *Biochem. J.* **55**, 35P.

Hall, D. A. (1954). "Old Age in the Modern World" (Ed. Tunbridge, R. E.), p. 165. Edinburgh, Livingstone.

Hall, D. A. (1955). *Biochem. J.* **59**, 459.

Hall, D. A. (1956). *Experientia Suppl.* **4**, 19.

Hall, D. A. (1957). *Gerontologia*, **1**, 347.

Hall, D. A. (1958). *In* "Connective Tissue" (Ed. Tunbridge, R. E.), p. 238. Oxford, Blackwell.

Hall, D. A. (1959). *Int. Rev. Cytol.* **8**, 211.

Hall, D. A. (1961a). *Biochem. J.* **78**, 49.

Hall, D. A. (1961b). *J. Atheroscler Res.* **1**, 173.

Hall, D. A. (1962). *Arch. Biochem. Suppl.* **1**, 239.

Hall, D. A. (1964). "Elastolysis and Ageing". Springfield, C. C. Thomas.

Hall, D. A. (1966). *Biochem. J.* **101**, 29.

Hall, D. A. (1967). *In* "Biological Aspects of Ageing" (Ed. Woolhouse, H.), p. 101. Cambridge University Press.

Hall, D. A. (1968a). *Exptl. Gerontol.* **3**, 77.

Hall, D. A. (1968b). *Gerontologia*, **14**, 97.

Hall, D. A. (1969a). *In* "Aging Life Processes" (Ed. Bakerman, S.), p. 79. Springfield, C. C. Thomas.

Hall, D. A. (1969b). Proc. 8th Inter. Congr. Gerontol., 113.

Hall, D. A. (1970a). *Gerontologia*, **16**, 325.

Hall, D. A. (1970b). *Nature, London*, **228**, 1314.

Hall, D. A. (1971). *In* "Biophysical Properties of the Skin" (Ed. Elden, H. R.), p. 187. New York, Wiley-Interscience.

Hall, D. A. (1972). *Age and Ageing*, **1**, 141.

Hall, D. A. (1973a). *In* "Textbook of Geriatric Medicine and Gerontology" (Ed. Brocklehurst, J. C.), p. 17. Edinburgh, Churchill, Livingstone.

Hall, D. A. (1973b). *Modern Geriatrics*, **3**, 26.

Hall, D. A. (1976a). *Arthritis and Rheumatism Res.* In Press.

Hall, D. A. (1976b). *In* "An Introduction to Bio-Mechanics of Joints and Joint Replacements" (Eds Dowson, D. and Wright, V.). Amsterdam, Elsevier.

Hall, D. A., Alderson, A. and Murray-Leslie, C. (1975). In Press.

Hall, D. A. and Czerkawski, J. W. (1959). *Biochem. J.* **73**, 356.

Hall, D. A. and Czerkawski, J. W. (1962). *In* "Collagen" (Ed. Ramanathan, N.), p. 419. New York, Wiley-Interscience.

Hall, D. A. and El-Ridi, S. (1976a). *In* "Methodology of Connective Tissue Research" (Ed. Hall, D. A.), p. 283. Oxford, Joynson-Bruvvers.

Hall, D. A. and El-Ridi, S. (1976b). *Trans. Biochem. Soc.* In Press.

Hall, D. A. and Gardiner, J. E. (1955). *Biochem. J.* **59**, 465.

Hall, D. A., Keech, M. K., Reed, R., Saxl, H., Tunbridge, R. E. and Wood, M. J. (1955). *J. Gerontol.* **10**, 388.

Hall, D. A., Lloyd, P. F., Saxl, H. and Happey, F. (1958). *Nature, London*, **181**, 1.

Hall, D. A., Lloyd, P. F., Saxl, H. and Happey, F. (1960). *Proc. Roy. Soc. B.* **151**, 497.

Hall, D. A. and the late W. A. Loeven (1975). Unpublished results.

Hall, D. A. and Reed, F. B. (1973). *Age and Ageing*, **2**, 218.

Hall, D. A., Reed, F. B., Nuki, G. and Vince, J. D. (1974). *Age and Ageing*, **3**, 15.

Hall, D. A., Reed, R. and Tunbridge, R. E. (1952). *Nature, London*, **170**, 264.

Hall, D. A., Reed, R. and Tunbridge, R. E. (1955). *Experimental Cell Res.* **8**, 35.

Hall, D. A. and Saxl, H. (1960). *Nature, London*, **187**, 547.

Hall, D. A. and Saxl, H. (1961). *Proc. Roy. Soc. B.* **155**, 202.

Hall, D. A. and Slater, R. S. (1973). *Age and Ageing*, **2**, 80.

Hall, D. A., Slater, R. S. and Tesal, I. S. (1973). *In* "Connective Tissue and Ageing" (Ed. Vogel, H. G.), p. 47. Amsterdam, Excerpta Medica.

Hall, D. A. and Tesal, I. S. (1976). *In* "Methodology of Connective Tissue Research" (Ed. Hall, D. A.), p. 181. Oxford, Joynson-Bruvvers.

Hall, D. A. and Tunbridge, R. E. (1957). *4th Internat. Congr. Gerontol., Merano*, **1**, 252.

Hall, D. A., Tunbridge, R. E. and Wood, G. C. (1953). *Nature, London*, **172**, 1099.

Halpern, B. N., Morard, J. C., Juster, M., Robert, L., Abadie, A. and Coudert, A. (1965). *Ann. N.Y. Acad. Sci.* **124**, 395.

Happey, F., Horton, W. G., McRae, T. P. and Naylor, A. (1955). *Nature, London*, **175**, 1032.

Happey, F., Naylor, A., Palframan, J., Pearson, C. H., Render, R. M. and Turner, R. L. (1974). *In* "Connective Tissues – Biochemistry and Pathophysiology" (Eds Fricke, R. and Hartmann, F.), p. 67. Berlin, Springer Verlag.

Harding, J. J. (1965). *Adv. Prot. Chem.* **20**, 109.

Harkness, R. D. (1968). *In* "Treatise on Collagen" (Ed. Gould, B. S.), Vol. 2, p. 247. New York, Academic Press.

Harkness, M. L. R., Harkness, R. D. and McDonald, D. A. (1957). *Proc. Roy. Soc. B.* **146**, 541.

Harkness, R. D., Marko, A. M., Muir, H. M. and Neuberger, A. (1954). *Biochem. J.* **56**, 558.

Harris, E. Jr and Sjoerdsma, A. (1966). *Lancet*, **ii**, 707.

Hascall, V. C. and Sajdera, S. W. (1969). *J. Biol. Chem.* **244**, 2384.

Hass, G. M. (1943). *Arch. Path.* **35**, 29.

Hauss, H. W., Junge-Hülsing, G. and Gerlach, U. (1968). "Die Unspeziefische Mesenchymreaktion". Stuttgart, Thieme Verlag.

Hayflick, L. (1965). *Exptl. Cell. Res.* **37**, 614.

Hayflick, L. (1970). *Exptl. Geront.* **5**, 291.

Haythorne, S. R., Taylor, F. A., Grego, H. W. and Barrier, A. Z. (1936a). *Am. J. Path.* **12**, 283.

Haythorne, S. R., Taylor, F. A., Grego, H. W. and Barrier, A. Z. (1936b). *Am. J. Path.* **12**, 303.

Heikkinen, E. (1968). *Acta. Physiol. Scand.* **74**, Suppl. 317, 1.

Heikkinen, E. (1969). *Scand. J. Clin. Lab. Invest.* **23**, Suppl. 108, 6.

Heikkinen, E. (1973). *In* "Frontiers of Matrix Biology. 1. Ageing of Connective Tissues. Skin" (Eds Robert, L. and Robert, B.), p. 107. Basel, Karger.

Heikkinen, E., Aalto, M., Viharsaari, T. and Kulonen, E. (1971). *J. Gerontol.* **26**, 294.

Heikkinen, E. and Juva, K. (1968). Abst. 5th Meet. Fed. Rurop. Biochem Socs. Prague, Abst. No. 561.

Heikkinen, E. and Kulonen, E. (1964). *Experientia*, **20**, 310.

Heikkinen, E. and Kulonen, E. (1968). *Biochim. Biophys. Acta.* **160**, 464.

Henneman, P. H. and Wallach, S. (1957). *Arch. Intern. Med.* **100**, 715.

Highberger, J. H., Gross, J. and Schmitt, O. (1950). *J. Amer. Chem. Soc.* **72**, 3321.

Hill, W. R. and Montgomery, H. (1940). *J. Invest. Dermatol.* **3**, 231.

Hilz, H., Erich, C. and Glaubitt, D. (1963). *Klin. Wschr.* **41**, 332.

Hoare, D. G. (1972). *Nature, London*, **236**, 437.

Hodge, A. J. and Petrushka, J. A. (1963). 5th Internat. Conf. on Electron Microscopy (Ed. Breese, S. S. Jr), Paper, QQ–1. New York, Academic Press.

Hoffman, A. S., Grande, L. A., Gibson, P., Park, J. B., Daly, C. H., Bornstein, P. and Ross, R. (1974). "Prospectives in Bioengineering". In Press.

Hoffman, P., Linker, A. and Meyer, K. (1956). *Science*, **124**, 1252.

Holliday, R. (1972). *Humangenetik*, **16**, 83.

Holliday, R. and Tarrant, G. M. (1972). *Nature, London*, **238**, 26.

Holman, R. L. (1961). *Amer. J. Clin. Nutr.* **9**, 565.

Holmes-Spicer, W. T. (1919). *Amer. J. Ophthalmol.* **2**, 340.

Hondius-Boldingh, W. and Laurence, E. B. (1968). *Eur. J. Biochem.* **5**, 191.

Houck, J. C. (1971). Personal communication. Quoted in Bullough (1973).

Howell, T. H. (1970). "A Student's Guide to Geriatrics". London, Staples Press.

Howes, E. L., Arandilla, J. A., Herbert, G. and Mandl, I. (1962). *J. Surg. Res.* **2**, 95.

Huble, J. (1957). *Acta. Endocrinol.* **25**, 59.

Hult, A. M. and Goltz, R. W. (1965). *J. Invest. Dermatol.* **44**, 408.

Hunter, J. A. A. and Finlay, B. (1973). *Internat. Revs. Connective Tissue Res.* **6**, 217.

Iverius, P. H. (1973). *In* "Atherogenesis: Initiating Factors", *Ciba Foundation Symposium*, **12**, 185.

Jackson, D. S. (1968). *In* "Repair and Regeneration" (Eds Winkle, N. von and Dunphy, J. E.), p. 161. New York, McGraw-Hill.

Jackson, D. S. (1973a). *In* "Connective Tissue and Ageing" (Ed. Vogel, H. G.), p. 191. Amsterdam Excerpta Medica.

Jackson, D. S. (1973b). *In* "Connective Tissue and Ageing" (Ed. Vogel, H. G.), p. 208. Amsterdam, Excerpta, Medica.

Jackson, D. S. and Bentley, J. P. (1968). *In* "Treatise on Collagen" (Ed. Gould, B. S.), p. 189. New York, Academic Press.

Jansen, L. H. and Rottier, P. B. (1957). *Dermatologica*, **115**, 106.

Jagenburg, O. R. (1959). *Scand. J. Clin. Lab. Invest.* **11**, Suppl. 43.

Jeanloz, R. W. (1960). *Arthritis and Rheumatism*, **3**, 233.

Joseph, K. T. and Gowri, C. (1970). *J. Sci. Industr. Res.* **24**, 504.

Jowsey, J. (1960). *Clin. Orthop.* **17**, 210.

Jowsey, J. (1966). *In* "Calcified Tissues" (Ed. Fleisch), p. 67. Berlin, Springer Verlag.

Junge-Hülsing, G. and Wagner, H. (1969). *In* "Ageing of Connective and Skeletal Tissue" (Eds Engel, A. and Larson, T.), p. 213. Stockholm, Nordiska Bokhandelsforlag.

Kadar, A., Robert, B. and Robert, L. (1973). *Pathol. Biol.* **21**, 80.

Kanabrocki, E. L., Fels, I. G. and Kaplan, E. (1960). *J. Gerontol.* **15**, 383.

Kang, A. H. (1972). *Biochemistry*, **11**, 1828.

Kao, K. T., Hilker, D. A. and McGavack, T. H. (1960). *Proc. Soc. Exptl. Biol. Med.* **104**, 359.

Kaplan, K. and Meyer, K. (1960). *Proc. Soc. Exptl. Biol. Med.* **105**, 78.

Keech, M. K. (1954a). *Yale J. Biol. Med.* **26**, 527.

Keech, M. K. (1954b). *Anat. Record.* **119**, 139.

Keech, M. K. (1955). *Ann. Rheum. Dis.* **14**, 19.

Keech, M. K. (1961). *J. Biophys. Biochem. Cytol.* **9**, 193.

Keech, M. K. and Reed, R. (1957). *Ann. Rheum. Dis.* **16**, 198.

Keech, M. K., Reed, R. and Wood, M. J. (1956). *J. Pathol. Bacteriol.* **71**, 477.

Keeley, F. W., Labella, F. S. and Queen, G. (1969). *Biochem. Biophys. Res. Commun.* **34**, 156.

Kefalides, N. A. (1969). Proc. 6th Congr. Intern. Diabetes Fed. Stockholm, p. 307.

Keiser, H. R., Gill, J. R., Sjoerdsma, A. and Bartter, F. C. (1964). *J. Clin. Invest.* **43**, 1073.

Kendall, E. G., Slocumb, C. H. and Polley, H. F. (1949). *Mayo Clinic*, **24**, 181.

Kennedi, R. M., Gibson, T. and Daly, C. H. (1965.) *In* "Biomechanics and Related Bioengineering Topics", p. 147. London, Pergamon Press.

Kirk, E. J. (1959). *Ann. N.Y. Acad. Sci.* **72**, 1006.

Kissmeyer, A. and With, C. (1922). *Brit. J. Dermatol.* **4**, 175.

Kivirikko, K. I. (1970). *Internat. Rev. Connective Tissue Res.* **5**, 93.

Kivirikko, K. I., Shudo, K., Sakaibara, S. and Prockop, D. J. (1972). *Biochemistry*, **11**, 122.

Kokas, E., Földes, I. and Banga, I. (1951). *Acta. Phys. Acd. Sci. Hung.* **2**, 333.

Kornfeld, S., Kornfeld, R., Neufeld, E. F. and O'Brien, P. J. (1964). *Proc. Nat. Acad. Sci. Wash.* **52**, 371.

Kowalewski, K. and Morrison, R. T. (1957). *Canadian J. Biochem. Physiol.* **35**, 771.

Kowalewski, K. (1958a). *Endocrinology*, **62**, 493.

Kowalewski, K. (1958b). *Endocrinology*, **63**, 759.

Kraemer, D. M. and Miller, H. (1953). *Arch. Pathol.* **55**, 70.

Kramsch, D. M. and Hollander, W. (1973). *J. Clin. Invest.* **52**, 236.

Kramsch, D. M., Franzblau, C. and Hollander, W. (1971). *J. Clin. Invest.* **50**, 1666.

Kramsch, D. M., Franzblau, C. and Hollander, W. (1974). *Adv. Exptl. Med. Biol.* **43**, 193.

Krafka, J. Jr (1937). *Arch. Path.* **23**, 1.

Kratky, O., Lauer, M. R., Retzenkofer, M. and Sekora, A. (1962). *In* "Collagen" (Ed. Ramanathan, N.), p. 227. New York, Wiley-Interscience.

Krohn, P. L. (1962). *Proc. Roy. Soc. B.* **157**, 128.

Labella, F. S. (1957). *Nature, London,* **180**, 1360.

Labella, F. S. (1962). *J. Gerontol.* **17**, 8.

Labella, F. S. (1971). *In* "Biophysical Properties of the Skin". (Ed. Elden, H. R.), p. 243. New York, Wiley-Interscience.

Labella, F. S. and Lindsay, W. G. (1963). *J. Gerontol.* **18**, 111.

Labella, F. S. and Vivian, S. (1967). *Biochem. Biophys. Acta.* **133**, 189.

Labella, F. S., Vivian, S. and Thornhill, D. P. (1966). *J. Gerontol.* **21**, 550.

Labella, F. S., Waykole, P. and Queen, G. (1968). *Biochim. Biophys. Res. Commun.* **30**, 333.

Labella, F. S., Keeley, F., Vivian, S. and Thornhill, D. (1967). *Biochim. Biophys. Res. Commun.* **26**, 748.

Laitinen, O. (1967). *Acta Endocrinol. Suppl.* **120**, p. 1.

Lamy, F., Craig, C. P. and Tauber, S. (1961). *J. Biol. Chem.* **236**, 86.

Langer, K. (1861). *S. Ber. Akad. Wiss. Abt. 1,* **44**, 19.

Lansing, A. I. (1954a). Symposium on Atherosclerosis. Nat. Acad. Sci. Nat. Res. Council, p. 50.

Lansing, A. I. (1954b). *Ciba Foundation Colloquia on Ageing,* **1**, 88.

Lansing, A. I. (1959). *In* "Connective Tissue. Thrombosis and Atherosclerosis (Ed. Page, I. H.), p. 167. New York, Academic Press.

Lansing, A. I., Alex, M. and Rosenthal, T. B. (1950a). *J. Gerontol.* **5**, 314.

Lansing, A. I., Rosenthal, T. B. and Alex, M. (1950b). *J. Gerontol.* **5**, 386.

Lansing, A. I., Blumenthal, H. T. and Gray, S. H. (1948). *J. Gerontol.* **3**, 87.

Lansing, A. I., Cooper, Z. K. and Rosenthal, T. B. (1953). *Anat. Record.* **115**, 340.

Lansing, A. I., Roberts, E., Ramasarma, G. B., Rosenthal, T. B. and Alex, M. (1951). *Proc. Soc. Exptl. Biol. Med.* **78**, 714.

Lapiccirella, R., Ferrari, C., Marrama, P. and Morini, C. (1960a). *Giorn. Gerontol.* **8**, 879.

Lapiccirella, R., Marrama, P., di Marco, G., Alberini, B. and Ferrari, C. (1960b). *Giorn. Gerontol.* **8**, 609.

Lapierre, C. M., Lemaers, A. and Kohn, L. D. (1971). *Proc. Natl. Acad. Sci. U.S.A.* **68**, 3054.

Lapierre, M., Lemaers, A. and Pierard, G. (1973). *In* "Biology of the Fibroblast" (Eds Kulonen, E. and Pikkarainen, J.), p. 379. London, Academic Press.

Laurent, T. C. (1970). *In* "Chemistry and Molecular Biology of the Intercellular Matrix" (Ed. Balazs, F. A.), p. 703. London, Academic Press.

Lazarides, E. L. and Lukens, L. N. (1971). *Nature, London*, **232**, 37.

Lazarus, G. S., Brown, R. S., Daniels, J. R. and Fullmer, H. M. (1968). *Science*, **159**, 1483.

Leary, T. (1941). *A.M.A. Arch. Pathol.* **32**, 507.

Lederer, J. and Bataille, J. R. (1969). *Ann. Endocrinol.* **30**, 598.

Ledvina, M. and Bartos, F. (1968). *Exptl. Gerontol.* **3**, 171.

Leighton, D. A. (1973). *In* "Textbook of Geriatric Medicine and Gerontology" (Ed. Brocklehurst, J. C.) p. 254. Edinburgh, Churchill, Livingstone.

Lenkiewicz, J. E., Davies, M. J. and Rosen, D. (1972). *Cardiovasc. Res.* **6**, 549.

Lent, R. and Franzblau, C. (1967). *Biochem. Biophys. Res. Commun.* **26**, 43.

Lent, R. W., Smith, B., Salcedo, L. L., Faris, B. and Franzblau, C. (1969). *Biochemistry*, **8**, 2837.

Leutert, G. (1964). *Morph. J.* **106**, 11.

Leutert, G. and Kreutz, W. (1964). *Mikr. Anat. Forsch.* **72**, 96.

Lev, M. and Sullivan, C. (1951). *Amer. J. Path.* **27**, 684.

Lev, M. and McMillan, J. B. (1961). *In* "Structural Aspects of Ageing" (Ed. Bourne, G. H.), p. 325. London, Pitman.

Levene, C. I. (1961). *J. Exptl. Med.* **114**, 295.

Levene, C. I. and Gross, J. (1959). *J. Exptl. Med.* **110**, 771.

Lewis, C. M. and Tarrant, G. M. (1972). *Nature, London*, **239**, 316.

Lewis, U. J., Williams, D. E. and Brink, N. G. (1956). *J. Biol. Chem.* **222**, 705.

Lindner, J. (1973). *In* "Connective Tissues and Ageing" (Ed. Vogel, H. G.), p. 119. Amsterdam, Excerpta Medica.

Lindner, J. and Johannes, G. (1973). *In* "Connective Tissue and Ageing" (Ed. Vogel, H. G.), p. 68. Amsterdam, Excerpta Medica.

Lindstedt, S. and Prockop, D. J. (1961). *J. Biol. Chem.* **236**, 1399.

Linke, K. W. (1955). *Z. Zellforsch.* **42**, 331.

Little, K. and Taylor, T. K. F. (1964). *In* "Age with a Future" (Ed. Hansen, P. F.), p. 311. Copenhagen, Munksgaard.

Little, K. and Valderrama, J. A. F. de (1968). *Gerontologia*, **4**, 109.

Lloyd, D. J. and Garrod, M. (1946). *J. Dyers, Col. Symp.* p. 24.

Loddi, L. and Maggi, L. (1953). *Acta Chir. Patavina*, **9**, 623.

Loeven, W. A. (1960). *Acta Physiol. Pharmacol. Neerl.* **9**, 44, 473.

Loeven, W. A. (1963). *Acta Physiol. Pharmacol. Neerl.* **11**, 350; **12**, 57.

Loeven, W. A. (1964). *Acta Physiol. Pharmacol. Neerl.* **12**, 497.

Loeven, W. A. (1965a). *In* "Structure and Function of Connective Tissue". N.A.T.O. Conference, p. 109. London, Butterworth.

Loeven, W. A. (1965b). *Acta Physiol. Pharmacol. Neerl.* **13**, 135.

Loeven, W. A. (1967). *Gerontologia*, **13**, 200.

Loeven, W. A. (1969). *J. Atheroscler. Res.* **9**, 35.

Loeven, W. A. and Baldwin, M. M. (1971a). *Gerontologia*, **17**, 170.

Loeven, W. A. and Baldwin, M. M. (1971b). *Gerontologia*, **17**, 203.

Loewi, G., Glynn, L. E. and Dorling, J. (1960). *J. Pathol. Bacteriol.* **80**, 1.

Lorenzen, I. (1959). *Proc. Soc. Exp. Biol. Med.* **102**, 453.

Lorenzen, I. (1962). *Acta Endocrinol.* **39**, 605, 615.

Lowry, O. H., Gilligan, D. R. and Katersky, E. M. (1941). *J. Biol. Chem.* **139**, 795.

Ludwig, A. W., Boas, N. F. and Soffer, L. J. (1950). *Proc. Soc. Exptl. Biol. Med.* **73**, 137.

McConkey, B., Fraser, G. M. and Bligh, A. S. (1965). *Ann. Rheum. Dis.* **24**, 219.

McConkey B., Fraser, G. M., Bligh, A. S. and Whiteley, H. (1963). *Lancet*, **i**, 693.

McConkey, B., Walton, K. W., Carney, S. A., Lawrence, J. C. and Ricketts, C. R. (1967). *Ann. Rheum. Dis.* **26**, 219.

McGavack, T. H. and Kao, K.-Y. T. (1960). *Exptl. Med. Surg.* **18**, 104.

McKusick, V. A. (1966). "Heritable Disorders of Connective Tissue", 3rd ed. St. Louis, C. V. Mosby.

McMillan, J. B. and Lev, M. (1962). *In* "Biological Aspects of Aging" (Ed. Shock, N. W.), p. 163. New York, Columbia University Press.

Maggi, V., Chayen, J., Gahan, P. B. and Brander, W. (1964). *Exp. Mol. Path.* **3**, 413.

Mandel, P. (1961). *Trans. 5th Internat. Conr. Angiol.* p. 25.

Mandl, I. (1961). *Advances in Enzymology*, **23**, 163.

Manley, G., Mullinger, R. N. and Lloyd, P. H. (1969). *Biochem. J.* **114**, 89.

Mark, H. and Susich, G. von (1924). *Z. Phys. Chem.* **4**, 431.

Martin, G. R. (1972). *In* "The Comparative Molecular Biology of Extracellular Matrices" (Ed. Slavkin, H. C.), p. 297. New York, Academic Press.

Martin, G. R. and Pinnell, S. R. (1968). *Proc. Internat. Symp. Como. Excerpta Med. Int. Congr. Series*, **188**, 109.

Mathews, M. B. (1962). *Biochim. Biophys. Acta*, **58**, 92.

Mathews, M. B. (1965). *In* "Structure and Function of Connective and Skeletal Tissue" (Eds Filton-Jackson, S., Harkness, R. D., Partridge, S. M. and Tristram, G. R.), p. 181. London, Butterworths.

Mathews, M. B. (1967). *Biol. Rev.* **42**, 499.

Mathews, M. B. (1970). *In* "Chemistry and Molecular Biology of the Intercellular Matrix" (Ed. Balazs, A. E.), Vol. 2, p. 1155. New York, Academic Press.

Mathews, M. B. (1973). *In* "Connective Tissue and Ageing" (Ed. Vogel, H. G.), p. 151. Amsterdam, Excerpta Medica.

Mathews, M. B. and Glagov, S. (1966). *J. Clin. Invest.* **45**, 1103.

Mathews, M. B. and Hinds, L. de C. (1963). *Biochim. Biophys. Acta*, **74**, 198.

Maximow, A. A. and Bloom, W. (1953). "Text Book of Histology". Philadelphia, Saunders.

Mechanic, J. and Levy, M. (1959). *J. Amer. Chem. Soc.* **81**, 1889.

Meema, H. E., Sheppard, R. H. and Rappaport, A. (1964). *Radiology*, **82**, 411.

Melcher, A. M. (1969). *Gerontologia*, **15**, 217.

Mercer, E. H. (1962). *Brit. Med. Bull.* **18**, 187.

Meyer, K. and Chaffee, E. (1941). *J. Biol. Chem.* **138**, 491.

Meyer, A. (1931). *Kinderheilk.* **50**, 596.

Meyer, J., Spier, F. and Neuwelt, F. (1940). *Arch. Intern. Med.* **65**, 171.

Miall, W. E., Ashcroft, M. T., Lovell, H. G. and Moore, F. (1967). *Hum Biol.* **39**, 445.

Milch, R. A. (1963). *Gerontologia*, **7**, 129.

Milch, R. A. (1965). *Monographs in Surg. Sci.* **2**, 261.

Miller, A. and Wray, J. S. (1971). *Nature, London*, **230**, 437.

Miller, E. J. (1976). *In* "Methodology of Connective Tissue Research" (Ed. Hall, D. A.), p. 197. Oxford, Joynson-Bruvvers.

Miller, E. J. and Fullmer, H. M. (1966). *J. Exptl. Med.* **123**, 1097.

Miller, E. J., Martin, G. R. and Piez, K. A. (1964). *Biochem. Biophys. Res. Commun.* **17**, 248.

Miller, E. J., Martin, G. R., Mecca, C. E. and Piez, K. A. (1965). *J. Biol. Chem.* 1965.

Miller, H., Haft, H. and Kraemer, D. (1952). *Proc. Soc. Exptl. Biol. Med.* **79**, 411.

Miller, H., Hirschman, A. and Kraemer, D. M. (1953). *Arch. Path.* **56**, 607.

Miller, W. R. (1971). Ph.D. Thesis, Leeds University.

Miller, W. R., Teale, J. D. and Davies, T. (1970). *Biochem. J.* **117**, 38.

Mills, B. G. and Bavetta, L. A. (1966). *J. Gerontol.* **21**, 449.

Montfort, I. and Perez-Tamayo, R. (1962). *Lab. Invest.* **11**, 463.

Moon, H. D. and Rinehart, J. F. (1952). *Circulation,* **6**, 481.

Morgan, D. B. and Newton-John, H. F. (1969). *Gerontologia,* **15**, 140.

Morgan, F. R. (1960). *J. Soc. Leather Trades Chem.* **44**, 170.

Morrison, R. I. G. (1970). *In* "Chemistry and Molecular Biology of the Intercellular Matrix" (Ed. Balazs, E. A.), Vol. 3, p. 1683. London, Academic Press.

Murray, M., Schrodt, G. R. and Berg, H. G. (1966). *Arch. Pathol., Chicago.* **82**, 138.

Mussini, E., Hutton, J. J. and Udenfriend, S. (1967). *Science,* **157**, 927.

Nemetschek, T. (1970). "Altern und Entwicklung". Stuttgart, Schattauer.

Neuberger, A., Perrone, J. C. and Slack, H. G. B. (1951). *Biochem. J.* **49**, 199.

Neuman, R. E. (1949). *Arch. Biochem.* **24**, 289.

Neuman, R. E. and Logan, M. A. (1950). *J. Biol. Chem.* **186**, 549.

Newman, D. L., Gosling, R. G. and Bowden, N. L. (1971). *Atherosclerosis,* **14**, 231.

Niehans, P. (1954). "Cellular Therapy". Munich and Berlin, Urban and Schwarzenberg.

Nimni, M. E. (1966). *Arthritis Rheumat.* **9**, 526.

Nimni, M. E., Guia, E. de and Bavetta, L. A. (1966). *J. Invest. Dermatol.* **47**, 156.

Nimni, M. E., Guia, E. de and Bavetta, L. A. (1967). *Biochem. J.* **102**, 143.

Nordin, B. E. C. (1966). *Clin. Orthop.* **45**, 17.

Nordin, B. E. C., Aaron, J., Gallagher, J. C. and Horsman, A. (1972). *In* "Nutrition in Old Age", *Symposium of the Swedish Nutrition Foundation,* **10**, 77.

Nordin, B. E. C. and Horsman, A. (1970). *In* "Osteoporosis" (Ed. Barzel, U.). New York, Grune and Stratton.

Nordin, B. E. C., Smith, D. A., Stevens, J. A. and Swanson, L. (1965). *In* "Medicine in Old Age" (ed. Agate, J. N.), p. 5. London, Pitman.

O'Brien, D., Bergstedt, J., Butterfield, J., Ibbott, F. and Lubchenco, L. L. (1960). *Acta Paediat.* **49**, 258.

Odland, L. M., Warwick, K. P. and Esselbaugh, N. C. (1958). *Montana, Agric. Exptl. Station. Tech. Bull.* 534.

Okajima, S. (1957). *Acta Inst. Anat. Niigata,* **44**, 63.

Oken, D. E. and Boucek, R. J. (1957). *Circulation Res.* **5**, 357.

Orekhovich, B. N., Tustanovskii, A. A., Oreckhovich, K. D. and Plotnikova, N. E. (1948). *Biokhimiya,* **13**, 55.

Orgel, L. E. (1963). *Proc. Nat. Acad. Sci. Wash.* **49**, 517.

Partridge, S. M. and Davis, H. F. (1955). *Nature, London,* **165**, 62.

Partridge, S. M., Davis, H. F. and Adair, G. S. (1955). *Biochem. J.* **61**, 21.

Partridge, S. M., Elsden, D. F., Thomas, J., Dorfman, A., Fesler, A. and Ho, P. (1964). *Biochem. J.* **93**, 30c.

Pauling, L. and Corey, R. B. (1951). *Proc. Natl. Acad. Sci. U.S.* **37**, 236.

Paz, M. A., Gallop, P. M., Blumenfeld, O., Henson, E. and Seifter, S. (1971a). *Biochem. Biophys. Res. Commun.* **43**, 289.

Paz, M. A., Henson, E., Blumenfeld, O., Seifter, S. and Gallop, P. M. (1971b). *Biochem. Biophy. Res. Commun.* **44**, 1518.

Paz, M. A., Pereya, B., Gallop, P. M. and Seifter, S. (1974). *J. Mechanochem. Cell. Molil.* **2**, 231.

Pearce, C. W., Foot, N. C., Jordan, G. L., Lans, S. W. and Wantz, G. E. (1960). *Surg. Gyn. Obstet.* **3**, 274.

Pearl, R. and Pearl, R. D. (1934). "The Ancestry of the Long Lived". Baltimore, Johns Hopkins Press.

Pearson, C. H. (1970). Ph.D. Thesis, University of Leeds.

Petrushka, J. A. and Sandberg, L. B. (1968). *Biochem. Biophys. Res. Commun.* **33**, 222.

Pierce, J. A. and Ebert, R. V. (1965). *Thorax,* **20**, 469.

Pinnell, S. R. and Martin, G. R. (1968). *Proc. Nat. Acad. Sci. Wash.* **61**, 708.

Piez, K. A. (1968). *Ann. Rev. Biochem.* **37**, 547.

Pittman, J. A. (1962). *J. Amer. Geriat. Soc.* **10**, 10.

Pope, F. M. (1972). *Trans. St. John's Hosp. Dermatol. Soc.* **58**, 235.

Püschel, J. (1930). *Beitr. Pathol. Anat.* **84**, 123.

Radharakrushnan, V. M., Ramanathan, N. and Nayudama, Y. (1964). *Leather Sci.* **11**, 102.

Ramachandran, G. N. (1963). *Internat. Revs. Connective Tissue Res.* **1**, 127.

Ramachandran, G. N. (1967). "Treatise on Collagen", Vol. 1. London, Academic Press.

Ramachandran, G. N. and Kartha, G. (1955). *Nature, London,* **176**, 593.

Rasmussen, B. L., Bruenger, E. and Sandberg, L. B. (1975). *Anal. Biochem.* **64**, 225.

Rauterberg, J. and Kühn, K. (1968). *F.E.B.S. Letters,* **1**, 230.

Rauterberg, J. and Kühn, K. (1968). *Hoppe-Seyler's Z. Physiol. Chem.* **349**, 611.

Rauterberg, J., Timpl, R. and Furthmayer, H. (1972). *Europ. J. Biochem.* **27**, 230.

Reed, F. B. and Hall, D. A. (1974). *In* "Connective Tissues – Biochemistry and Pathophysiology" (Eds Fricke, R. and Hartmann, F.), p. 290. Berlin, Springer Verlag.

Reed, R. (1957). *In* "Connective Tissue" (Ed. Tunbridge, R. E.), p. 299, Oxford, Blackwell.

Reed, R. (1973). *In* "Internat. Rev. Connect. Tissue. Res. VI" (Eds Hall, D. A. and Jackson, D. S.), p. 257. New York, Academic Press.

Reed, R., Wood, M. J. and Keech, M. K. (1956). *Nature, London,* **177**, 697.

Rhodin, J. and Dalham, T. (1955). *Exptl. Cell Res.* **9**, 371.

Rich, A. and Crick, F. H. C. (1955). *Nature, London,* **176**, 915.

Rich, A. and Crick, F. H. C. (1958). *In* "Recent Advances in Glue and Gelatin Research" (Ed. Stainsby, G.), p. 20. New York, Pergamon Press.

Rich, A. and Crick, F. H. C. (1961). *J. Mol. Biol.* **3**, 483.

Ridge, M. D. and Wright, V. (1964). *Biorheology,* **2**, 67.

Ridge, M. D. and Wright, V. (1965a). *In* "Biomechanics and Related Bio-engineering Topics" (Ed. Kennedi, R. M.), p. 165. Oxford, Pergamon Press.

Ridge, M. D. and Wright, V. (1965b). *Brit. J. Derm.* **77**, 639.

Ridge, M. D. and Wright, V. (1966a). *Gerontologia,* **12**, 174.

Ridge, M. D. and Wright, V. (1966b). *J. Invest. Dermatol.* **46**, 341.

Rigby, B. J. (1964). *Nature, London,* **202**, 1072.

Rigby, C. J., Hirai, N., Spikes, J. D. and Eyring, H. (1959). *J. Gen. Physiol.* **43**, 265.

Rinderknecht, H., Geokas, M. C., Silverman, P. and Haverback, B. J. (1968). *Clin. Chem. Acta,* **19**, 89.

Roach, M. R. and Burton, A. C. (1957). *Canadian J. Biochem Physiol.* **35**, 681.

Roach, M. R. and Burton, A. C. (1959). *Canadian J. Biochem. Physiol.* **37**, 557.

Robert, L. and Samuel, P. (1957). *Ann. Biol. Clin., Paris*, **15**, 453.

Robert, L. and Samuel, P. (1957). *Experientia*, **13**, 167.

Robert, L., Derouette, S. and Moczar, E. (1971). *Gerontologia*, **17**, 65.

Robert, B., Szigeti, M., Derouette, J. C., Robert, L., Biosson, H. and Fabre, M. T. (1971). *Europ. J. Biochem.* **21**, 507.

Robins, S. P. and Bailey, A. J. (1973). *F.E.B.S. Letters*, **33**, 167.

Robins, S. P., Shimokomaki, M. and Bailey, A. J. (1973). *Biochem. J.* **131**, 771.

Rodén, L. (1970). *In* "Chemistry and Molecular Biology of the Intercellular Matrix" (Ed. Balazs, E. A.), Vol. 2, p. 797. New York, Academic Press.

Rodin, E. L., Swann, D. A. and Weiser, P. A. (1970). *Nature, London*, **228**, 377.

Rollhauser, H. (1950). *Gegenbaurs. Morphol. Jahrb.* **90**, 249.

Rosenberg, L., Hellmann, W. and Kleinschmidt, A. K. (1970). *J. Biol. Chem.* **245**, 4123.

Roseberry, H. H., Hastings, A. B. and Morse, J. K. (1931). *J. Biol. Chem.* **90**, 395.

Ross, R. (1973). *J. Histochem.* **21**, 199.

Ross, R. and Benditt, E. P. (1964). *J. Cell. Biol.* **22**, 365.

Ross, R. and Bornstein, P. (1969). *J. Cell. Biol.* **40**, 366.

Rychewaert, A., Parot, S. and Tamisier, S. (1967). *Rev. Fr. Elud. Clin. Biol.* **12**, 803.

Salmon, W. D. Jr, Bowes, P. H. and Thompson, E. Y. (1963). *J. Lab. Clin. Med.* **61**, 120.

Salvini, L. (1960). *Giorn. Gerontol.* **8, 551.**

Sams, W. M. and Smith, J. G. (1961). *J. Invest. Dermatol.* **37**, 447.

Sandberg, L. B. (1975). *Internat. Revs. Connective Tissue Res.* **7**, 160.

Sanders, H. J. (1972). *Chem. Eng. News*, July, p. 13.

Sandson, J. and Hamerman, D. (1962). *J. Clin. Invest.* **41**, 1817.

Sanwald, R., Ritz, E. and Wiese, G. (1971). *Atherosclerosis*, **13**, 247.

Saxl, H. (1957a). Proc. 4th Internat. Congr. Gerontol. Merans., p. 67.

Saxl, H. (1957b). *Gerontologia*, **1**, 142.

Saxl, H. (1961). *J. Roy. Microscop. Soc.* **79**, 319.

Saxl, H. and Hall, D. A. (1967). *In* "Cowdry's Atherosclerosis", 2nd ed. (Ed. Blumenthal, H. T.), p. 141. Springfield, C. C. Thomas.

Scarselli, V. (1959). *Nature, London*, **184**, 1565.

Scarselli, V. (1960). *Giorn. Biochem.* **9**, 153.

Scarselli, V., Chierichetti, P. and Pelizzati, P. (1960). *Boll. Soc. Ital. Biol. Sper.* **36**, 1865.

Schaub, M. C. (1964). *Helv. Physiol. Acta*, **22**, C 38.

Schmitt, F. O., Hall, C. E. and Jakus, M. E. (1942). *J. Cellular Comp. Physiol.* **20**, 11.

Schmitt, O., Gross, J. and Highberger, J. H. (1953). *Proc. Natl. Acad. Sci. U.S.* **39**, 459.

Schmitt, W. and Beneke, G. (1971). *In* "Molekulare und Zelluläre Aspekte des Alterns" (Eds Platt, D. and Lasch, H. G.), p. 37. Stuttgart, Schaltauer.

Schneider, R. R., Walford, R. L. and Dignan, W. J. (1960). *J. Appl. Physiol.* **15**, 992

Schroeder, W. A., Honen, L. and Green, F. C. (1953). *Proc. Nat. Acad. Sci. U.S.* **39**, 23.

Schwarz, W. (1957). *In* "Connective Tissue" (Ed. Tunbridge, R. E.), p. 144. Oxford, Blackwell.

Schwarz, W. (1961). *In* "Structure of the Eye" (Ed. Smelser, G. K.), p. 283. New York, Academic Press.

Sedlin, E. D. (1965). *Acta Orthopt. Scand.* **36,** Suppl. 83, p. 1.

Serafini-Fracassini, A. and Tristram, G. R. (1966). *Proc. Roy. Soc. B.* **59,** 334.

Serafini-Fracassini, A., Field, J. M., Rodger, G. W. and Spina, M. (1975). In Press.

Sheppard, R. H. and Meema, H. E. (1967). *Ann. Intern. Med.* **66,** 531.

Shields, C. S., Coulson, W. F., Kimball, D. A., Carnes, W. H., Cartwright, G. E. and Wintrobe, M. M. (1962). *Amer. J. Pathol.* **41,** 603.

Shimizu, M. (1955). *C.R. Soc. Biol., Paris,* **149,** 853.

Shock, N. W. (1964). *In* "Age with a Future" (Ed. Hansen, P. F.), p. 13. Copenhagen, Munksgaard.

Shulman, H. J. and Meyer, K. (1968). *J. Exptl. Med.* **128,** 1353.

Shuster, S. and Bottoms, E. (1963). *Clin. Sci.* **25,** 487.

Shuster, S. and Bottoms, E. (1966). *Nature, London,* **214,** 599.

Siegel, R. C., Pinnell, S. R. and Martin, G. R. (1970). *Biochemistry,* **9,** 4486.

Silberberg, R. and Lesker, P. A. (1973). *In* "Connective Tissue and Ageing" (Ed. Vogel, H. G.), p. 98. Amsterdam, Excerpta Medica.

Silpananta, P., Dunstone, J. R. and Ogston, A. G. (1968). *Biochem. J.* **109,** 43.

Sippel, T. O. (1965). *Invest. Ophthalmol.* **44,** 423.

Slater, R. S. (1966). Ph.D. Thesis, University of Leeds.

Slater, R. S. and Hall, D. A. (1973). *In* "Connective Tissue and Ageing" (Ed. Vogel H. G.), p. 241. Amsterdam, Excerpta Medica.

Smith, D. W., Weissman, N. and Carnes, W. H. (1968). *Biochem. Biophys. Res. Commun.* **31,** 309.

Smith, E. B. (1965). *J. Atheroscler. Res.* **5,** 224.

Smith, E. B., Evans, P. H. and Downham, M. D. (1967). *J. Atheroscler. Res.* **7,** 171.

Smith, J. G. Jr, Davidson, E. A. and Clark, R. D. (1962a). *Nature, London,* **195,** 716.

Smith, J. G. Jr, Davidson, E. A., Sams, W. H. and Clark, R. D. (1962b). *Nature, London,* **195,** 716.

Smith, J. G. Jr, Sams, W. H., Davidson, E. A. and Clark, R. D. (1962c). *Arch. Dermatol.* **86,** 741.

Smith, J. W. (1968). *Nature, London,* **219,** 157.

Smith, P. (1883). *Trans. Ophthalm. Soc. U.K.* **3,** 79.

Spiro, R. G. and Fukushi, S. (1969). *J. Biol. Chem.* **244,** 2049.

Spiro, M. J. and Spiro, R. G. (1971). *J. Biol. Chem.* **246,** 4919.

Starcher, R. C., Partridge, S. M. and Elsden, D. F. (1967). *Biochem. J.* **6,** 2425.

Starling's Principles of Human Physiology (1941). (Ed. Lovatt Evans, C.), 8th ed., p. 387. London, Churchill.

Stein, W. H. and Miller, E. G. Jr (1938). *J. Biol. Chem.* **123,** 599.

Stein, Y. and Stein, O. (1973). *In* "Atherogenesis: Initiating Factors", *Ciba Foundation Symposium,* **12,** 165.

Steinach, E. (1920). "Rejuvenation through Experimental Restoration of Pubertal Glands". Berlin, Springer Verlag.

Stetten, M. R. (1949). *J. Biol. Chem.* **181,** 31.

Stetten, M. R. and Schoenheimer, R. (1944). *J. Biol. Chem.* **153,** 113.

Steven, F. S. (1964). *Ann. Rheum. Dis.* **23,** 300.

Steven, F. S. and Jackson, D. S. (1967). *Biochem. J.* **104,** 534.

Strehler, B. L. (1962). "Time, Cells and Aging". New York, Academic Press.

Stucke, K. (1950). *Chirurg.* **29,** 16.

Sykes, B. C. and Partridge, S. M. (1974). *Biochem. J.* **141,** 567.

Szabo, D. and Cseh, G. (1962). *Naturwiss,* **49,** 260.

Szirmai, J. A. (1970). *In* "Chemistry and Biology of the Intercellular Matrix" (Ed. Balazs, E. A.), p. 1279. London, Academic Press.

Tammes, A. R. (1964). *Lab. Invest.* **13**, 1234.

Tainenheim, E. G. von (1901). *Weiner, Klin. Wochenschr.* **14**, 1038.

Tanner, J. M. (1955). "Growth at Adolescence". Oxford, Blackwell.

Tanner, J. M. and Whitehouse, H. H. (1955). *Amer. J. Phys. Anthrop.* **13**, 743.

Tanzer, M. L. (1968). *J. Biol. Chem.* **243**, 4045.

Tanzer, M. L., Housley, T., Berube, L., Fairweather, R., Franzblau, C. and Gallop, P. M. (1973). *J. Biol. Chem.* **248**, 393.

Tattersall, R. N. and Savile, R. (1950). *Quart. J. Med.* **19**, 151.

Taubenhaus, M. and Amromin, G. D. (1950). *J. Lab. Clin. Med.* **36**, 7.

Taylor, N. W. and Sheard, C. (1929). *J. Biol. Chem.* **81**, 479.

Teale, J. D. (1971). Ph.D. Thesis, Leeds University.

Teale, J. D., Davies, T. and Hall, D. A. (1972). *Biochem. Res. Commun.* **42**, 234.

Tesal, S. I. (1971). Ph.D. Thesis, University of Leeds.

Tesal, S. I. and Hall, D. A. (1972). *Proc. 9th Internat. Congr. Gerontology. Kiev,* **2**, 58.

Thomas, J. and Partridge, S. M. (1960). *Biochem, J.* **74**, 600.

Thomas, J., Elsden, D. F. and Partridge, S. M. (1963). *Nature, London,* **200**, 651.

Tindel, S., Schneider, I. J., Shapiro, D. and State, D. (1962). *Nature, London,* **195**, 288.

Tolnay, P. and Bagdy, D. (1959). *Biochim. Biophys. Acta,* **31**, 566.

Tolnay, P., Solyom, A. and Borsy, J. (1962). *Naturwiss.* **49**, 259.

Traub, W. and Piez, K. A. (1971). *Adv. Prot. Chem.* **25**, 243.

Tregear, R. T. (1966). "Theoretical and Experimental Biology", Vol. V, p. 73. New York, Academic Press.

Tsiganos, C. P. and Muir, H. (1973). *In* "Connective Tissue and Ageing" (Ed. Vogel, H. G.), p. 132. Amsterdam, Excerpta Medica.

Tunbridge, R. E. (1958). "Connective Tissue". Oxford, Blackwell.

Tunbridge, R. E., Astbury, W. T., Tattersall, R. N., Reed, R., Eaves, G. and Hall, D. A. (1950).

Tunbridge, R. E., Tattersall, R. N., Hall, D. A., Astbury, W. T. and Reed, R. (1952). *Clinical Sci.* **11**, 315.

Tustanovsky, A. A., Zaides, A. L., Orlovskaja, G. V. and Mihajlor, H. N. (1954). *Dokl. Akad. Nauk. SSSR.* **97**, 191.

Tustanovsky, A. A., Zaides, A. L., Banga, I. and Orlovskaja, K. V. (1960). *Gerontologia,* **4**, 198.

Uitto, J. (1971). *Ann. Clin. Res.* **3**, 250.

Uitto, J., Halme, J., Hannuksela, M., Peltokallio, P. and Kivirikko, K. I. (1969). *Scand. J. Clin. Lab. Invest.* **23**, 241.

Unna, P. G. (1896). "Histopathological Diseases of the Skin" (Translater, Walker, N.), p. 984. New York, Macmillan.

Varadi, D. P. and Hall, D. A. (1965). *Nature, London,* **208**, 1224.

Veis, A. (1965). *Internat. Revs. Connective Tissue Res.* **3**, 113.

Veis, A. (1967). *In* "Treatise and Collagen" (Ed. Ramachandran, G. N.), p. 207 New York, Academic Press.

Veis, A. (1972). *In* "The Comparative Molecular Biology of Extracellular Matrices" (Ed. Slavkin, H. C.), p. 297. New York, Academic Press.

Veis, A. and Anesy, J. (1965). *J. Biol. Chem.* **240**, 3899.

Verzar, F. (1955). *Helv. Physiol Pharmacol. Acta,* **13**, 64.

Verzar, F. (1957). *Gerontologia,* **1**, 363.

Verzar, F. (1963). "Lectures on Experimental Gerontology". Springfield, C. C. Thomas.

Verzar, F. (1964). *Internat. Revs. Connective Tissue Res.* **2**, 244.

Verzar, F. and Hüber, K. (1958). *Acta Anat.* **33**, 215.

Verzar, F. and Meyer, A. (1959). *Gerontologia*, **3**, 184.

Verzar, F. and Spichtin, H. (1966). *Gerontologia*, **12**, 48.

Viidik, A. (1966a). *In* "Studies on the Anatomy and Function of Bone and Joints" (Ed. Evans, F. G.), p. 17. Berlin, Springer Verlag.

Viidik, A. (1966b). *Proc. 7th Internat. Congr. Gerontol.*, p. 173.

Viidik, A. (1968). *J. Biomech.* **1**, 3.

Viidik, A. (1972). *Z. Anat. Entw. Gesch.* **136**, 204.

Viidik, A. (1973). *Internat. Revs. Connective Tissue Res.* **6**, 127.

Viidik, A. and Ekholm, R. (1968). *Z. Anat. Entw. Gesch.* **127**, 154.

Viidik, A. and Mägi, M. (1967). "7th Int. Conf. on Med. And Biol. Engineering". p. 507. Stockholm, Almqvist and Wiksell.

Viljanto, J., Isomaki, H. and Kulonen, E. (1962). *Acta Endocrinol.* **41**, 395.

Viola, S., Citi, S., Leone, O., Salvini, L. and Grandonico, F. (1960). *Giorn. Gerontol.* **8**, 655.

Virchow, R. (1871). "Cellular Pathology and its Dependence on Physiological and Pathological Tissue Studies", p. 40. Berlin, Hirschwald.

Vogel, H. (1974). *Connective Tissue Res.* **2**, 177.

Voronoff, S. (1920). "Studies on Methods for Increasing Vital Energy and Prolonging Life". Paris, Grosset.

Voronoff, S. (1929). "Testicular Grafting from Ape to Man". London, Bretans.

Walford, R. L. and Schneider, R. (1959). *Proc. Soc. Exptl. Biol. Med.* **101**, 31.

Walford, R. L. and Sopher, R. (1966). *Lab. Invest.* **15**, 1248.

Walford, R. L., Carter, P. K. and Schneider, R. B. (1964). *AMA Arch. Path.* **78**, 43.

Walford, R. L., Hirose, F. M. and Doyle, P. (1959). *Lab. Invest.* **8**, 948.

Walker, D. G., Lapierre, C. M. and Gross, J. (1964). *Biochem. Biophys. Res. Commun.* **15**, 397.

Wegelius, O. and Knorring, J. von (1964). *Acta Med. Scand.* **175**, Suppl. 412, 233.

Weil, C., Frei, P., Weigel, W. and Kasinski, B. (1969). *Rev. Rheum.* **36**, 732.

Weinbach, E. C. and Garbus, J. (1956). *Nature, London*, **178**, 1225.

Weinbach, E. C. and Garbus, J. (1959). *J. Biol. Chem.* **234**, 412.

Wellman, W. E. and Edwards, J. E. (1950). *Arch. Pathol.* **50**, 183.

Wells, H. G. (1933). *In* "Arteriosclerosis. A Survey of the Problems" (Ed. Cowdry, E. V.), p. 323. New York, Macmillan.

Wertheim, H. G. (1847). *Chim. Phys.* **21**, 385.

Wilson, P. D. (1973). *Gerontologia*, **19**, 79.

Winter, K. K. and Frankel, S. (1956). *Fed. Proc.* **15**, 539.

Wirtschafter, Z. Y. and Bentley, J. P. (1962). *Lab. Invest.* **11**, 316.

Wolinsky, R. (1970). *Atherosclerosis*, **11**, 251.

Wolinsky, H. and Glagov, S. (1967). *Circulation Res.* **20**, 99.

Wolinsky, H. and Glagov, S. (1969). *Circulation Res.* **25**, 677.

Wolpers, C. (1944). *Klin. Wschr.* **23**, 169.

Wood, G. C. (1954). *Biochim. Biophys. Acta*, **15**, 311.

Wood, G. C. (1960). *Biochem. J.* **75**, 598.

Wood, G. C. (1964). *Internat. Revs. Connective. Res.* **2**, 1.

Woolf, L. I. and Norman, A. D. (1957). *J. Pediat.* **50**, 271.

Wright, V., Dowson, D. and Kerr, J. (1973). *Internat. Revs. Connective Tissue Res.* **6,** 106.

Wright, D. G. and Rennels, D. C. (1964). *J. Bone Jt. Surg.* **46,** 482.

Wyckoff, R. W. G. and Corey, R. B. (1936). *Proc. Soc. Exptl. Biol. Med.* **34,** 285.

Yamada, H. (1970). "Strength of Biological Materials". Baltimore, Williams and Wilkins.

Yu, S. Y. (1967). *In* Cowdry's "Arteriosclerosis" (Ed. Blumenthal, H. T.), 2nd ed., p. 170. Springfield, C. C. Thomas.

Yu, S. Y. (1970). *Anal. Biochem.* **37,** 212.

Yu, S. Y. (1971). *Lab. Invest.* **25,** 121.

Yu, S. Y. and Blumenthal, H. T. (1958). *J. Gerontol.* **13,** 316.

Yu, S. Y. and Blumenthal, H. T. (1963). *J. Gerontol.* **18,** 119.

Zorzoli, A. (1969). *In* "Ageing Life Processes" (Ed. Bakerman, S.), p. 52. Springfield, C. C. Thomas.

Ziff, M., Kibrick, A., Dresner, E. and Gribetz, H. J. (1956). *J. Clin. Invest.* **35,** 579.

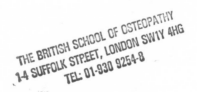

Index

Adventitia, 34
Age, biological, 1
  changes in collagen, 67, 69, 73, 93; in
    elastin, 95ff.; in glycosaminoglycans,
    141; in stature, 52
  chronological, 1
  phenomena, genetically determined, 3
    random, 4
Ageing, pathological, 173
  physiological, 173
  process, hormonal control of, 11
  theories, 1ff.
    molecular applications of, 9
Aldehydes, crosslinking by, 134
Aldimines, 88
Allysine, 90, 121
Allysine aldol, 90, 121
β-Amino propionitrile, 87
δ-Amino adipic acid semialdehyde, *see*
    allylysine
Anabolic steroids, 165
Androgen secretion, 156
Anisotropic fibres, 117
Aortic wall, 26ff.
  calcification of, 37
  calcium content, 100, 107
  changes in dimensions of, 27
  cellular changes in, 19
  collagen, 80
  elastic degeneration, 35
  elastic lamellae, 33
  elastic content, 102, 107, 111
  glycosaminoglycans, 20
  intima, 29
  lipoidoses, 177
  media, 31
  physical properties, 26
  pseudoelastin in, 38, 109, 117
  smooth muscle, 27
  ^{35}S-sulphate incorporation by, 20
  vasa vasorum, 34, 178
Arteries, repair processes in, 3, 174

Atherogenic index, 174
Atherosclerosis, 174ff.
Arteriosclerosis, 100

Biochemical changes with age, 79ff.
Biological age, 1
Bone, linkages in, 92
  loss, 55
  resorption, 52
  turnover, 55

Calcification, 37
Calcium, cross linkages, 11, 129
  in aortic wall, 101
  in elastolysis, 99
Cardiovascular disease, 174
  tissue, collagen in, 80
    elastin content, 95
    pseudoelastin in, 95
Cartilage, articular, 19, 57
  costal, 141
  glycosaminoglycans in, 141
  knee joint, 142
  linkages in, 92
  structure of, 58
Catabolic hormones, 169
Cataract, 65
Cells, 16–20
  daughter, 6, 145
  differentiation of, 13
  fall out, 10
  immortal, 5
  intrusive, 17
  mitotic division of, 5, 164
  mutation, 8
  pigmented, 17
  population changes with age, 17
Cellulose containing fibres, 117
Chalones, 164
Chelating agents, effect on elastolysis,
    130ff.
Chondroitin sulphates, 137

Chronological age, 1
Collagen, α-chains, 82
  biosynthesis, 86, 145
  bundles, 41
  cross-links in, 80ff.
  cross-striations, 71
  degradation with age, 73, 149
  diffraction pattern, 67
  fibre diameter, 70
  fine structure, 71
  hypophysectomy and, 167
  in vitro synthesis, 146
  molecular structure of, 81
  polymers, 85, 145
  structure, 81
  synthesis, 16, 70, 86, 147
  telopeptides, 82
Collagenase, *clostridial*, 74
  tissue, 149
Congo-red dyed elastin, 153
Costal cartilage, 141
Criteria of ageing, 2
Cross-links, age variations, 93
  in collagen, 85ff.
  in elastin, 121ff.
  lysine based, 87, 122
  sites of, 89
Cutis laxa, 116

Dehydro-dihydroxylysinonorleucine, 92
Dehydrolysinonorleucine, 124
Dermatan sulphate, 138
Dermis, *see* skin
Desmosines, 121–129
Differentiation, 13
Dihydroxynorleucine, 90
Dityrosine linkages, 135

Elastase,
  activity in aortic wall, 35, 156
  and atherosclerosis, 176
  cellular origins, 152
  in human pancreas, 133, 177
  in human plasma, 153, 157
  inhibition by chelating agents, 158; by
    human plasma, 158; by rat plasma,
    160
  multiple nature of, 100, 156
  in rat pancreas, 158
  secretion into circulation, 153

Elastic degradation, 35
  fibres, synthesis of, 16
  lamellae, 34
  stiffness, modulus of, 24
  tissue, microfibrils of, 75
Elastin, amino acid composition of, 96,
    106, 109, 111
  Congo-red dyed, 153
  content of tissues, 95, 107
  cross-links in, 121ff.
  diffraction pattern, 69
  fragmentation of, 174
  metabolism of, 167
  reduplication, 174
  sialic acid content, 133
  in skin, 103
Elastolipoprotein lipase, 163, 178
Elastolysis, 98
  activation by Ca EDTA, 133
  as a tool in tissue research, 100
  calcium and, 132
  co-ordinately bound calcium in, 99
  kinetic constants of, 99
  measurement of, 154
  velocity of, 101
Elastomucase, 163, 179
Embryonic tissues, 13
Enzymes, 10, 131, 149ff.
  apparent activity of, 10
  inhibitors of, 10
  tissue, 10, 17
Error theory, 7
Ester linkages, 94
Ethylene diamine tetraacetic acid, 130
Extracellular tissues, 21
Eye, 64

Fatty acids, 163
  streaks, 177
Fibroblasts, 16
  age changes in activity, 145
Fraction C, 91

Genes, 4
  de-represssion of, 5, 119
  repression of, 7
Glycosaminoglycans, 136ff.
  age changes, 141
  sulphate incorporation in, 149
  synthesis, 147

Glycoproteins, 94, 136
Glycosylamines, 93
Granuloma tissue, 146, 149
Growth velocity, 1

Height changes with age, 52
Histiocytes, 17
Hormonal control of enzyme activity, 11
  of tissue metabolism, 12, 164ff.
Hormones, anabolic, 164
  catabolic, 169
  female, sex, 169
Human plasma, elastase in, 153, 157
  elastase inhibitor in, 158
Hyaluronic acid, 137
Hydroxyallysine, 91
Hydroxynorleucine, 90
Hydroxyproline in urine, 150
  synthesis, 147
Hypertension, 174
Hypophysectomy, 167

Intermolecular linkages, 90
Intervertebral disc, 59
  collagen content of, 61
  fibrosis of, 60
  glycosaminoglycans of, 144
  moisture content, 61
  physical properties, 60
  structure, 59
Intima, calcium content, 100
  fragmentation with age, 31
  structure of, 29
Intramolecular linkages, 90

Keratin sulphate, 138
Knee joint cartilage, 142

Lathyrism, 87
Lifespan, 2
Ligamentum nuchae, 106, 133
Lipid accumulation by smooth muscle
  cells, 35
Lipolytic enzymes, 162
Lipoprotein lipase, 179
Longevity, 2
Life expectancy, 2
Lung, 63
Lysinonorleucine, 90, 124
Lysine hydroxylase, 147

Mast cells, 17
Mechanical stress, 116
Metabolism, 145ff.
Media, calcium content, 100
  structure of, 31
  tension/extension curves for, 33
Menopause, 2, 155
Merodesmosine, 121
Metacollagen, 23
Metallic cross-linkages, 136
Microfibrils of elastin, 112

Oestrogens, 167
Osteoporosis, 51ff.
  and catabolic hormones, 169
  oestrogens and, 167

Pancreas, elastase content, 133, 158, 177
Pathological ageing, 173
Physiological ageing, 173
Pituitary hormone, 167
Plasma,
  human, elastase in, 153, 157; elastase
    inhibitor in, 158
  rat, elastase inhibitor in, 160
Prednisolone and collagen metabolism,
  169
Pro-collagen, 86
  peptidase, 147
Programmed age theory, 4
Proline hydroxylase, 147
Proteoglycanases, 161
Proteoglycans, 136ff.
  polydispersity of, 139
Protocollagen, 86
Pseudoelastin, 73
  in aortic wall, 38, 117
  chemical composition of, 112
  in cellulose-containing fibres, 119
  group of, 75
  separation from tissue, 111
  in skin, 104, 105, 114, 115
  tinctorial properties, 108
Pseudopeptide linkages, 94
Pseudoxanthoma elasticum, 157
Pulmonary artery elastin, 107

Random error theory, 7
Rat plasma, elastase inhibitor in, 160
Remodelling of tissues, 149

Repair processes, 3, 174
RNA, messenger, 7
  transport, 7

Schiff's bases, 88, 124
Senescence, 2
Senile purpura, 42, 104
Sialic acid, 133
Skin, basophilic degeneration, 104
  collagen bundles, 41
  collagen content, 79
  effect of collagenase in, 105
  elastase extractable material in, 115
  elastica staining material in, 42, 103
  elastin content, 103, 114
  glycosaminoglycans in, 143
  linkages in, 92
  load/extension curves for, 46
  morphology in ageing, 42
  pseudoelastin in, 105
  staining properties, 43
  stiffness, 49
  structure, 40
  thickness, 79
  transplantation, 5
  ultra-violt irradiation, 45, 105
Smooth muscle cells, in aortic wall, 27
  differentiation, 34
  function of, 34
Steroids, anabolic, 165
  catabolic, 169
Stress, effect on tissues, 102

Tendon, contraction, 21
  glycoproteins in, 140
  models, 24

  stress/strain curves, 25
  tensile properties, 23
Theories of ageing, 1
Thyroid gland, age changes, 12
  atrophy, 166
Thyroid hormone, 166
Tissue, collagenases, 73, 113
  collagen content, 79
  elastosis, 73
  enzymes, 10
  linkages, 92
  macrostructure, 13ff.
  metabolism, 145ff.
    hormonal control of, 164
  remodelling, 149
Tissues, degenerate fibres in, 73
  elastin content of, 95
  embryonic, 13
  extracellular, 21
  microstructure of, 67ff.
  structural characteristics of, 13
Tropocollagen, 71, 82
  covalent linkages, 72
  denaturation, 83
  hydrogen bonds in, 81
  molecular weight, 71
Ultra-violet irradiation of skin, 45, 105

Vasa vasorum, 34, 178
Vascular disease, 174ff.
Vocal cords, 166

X-ray diffraction patterns, 57

Young's modulus, 23, 47